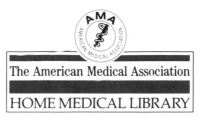

The American Medical Association

HOME MEDICAL LIBRARY

ACCIDENTS AND EMERGENCIES

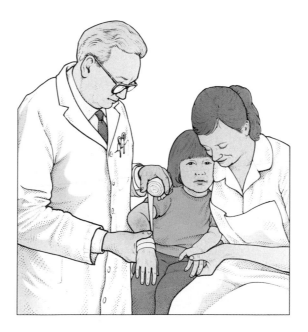

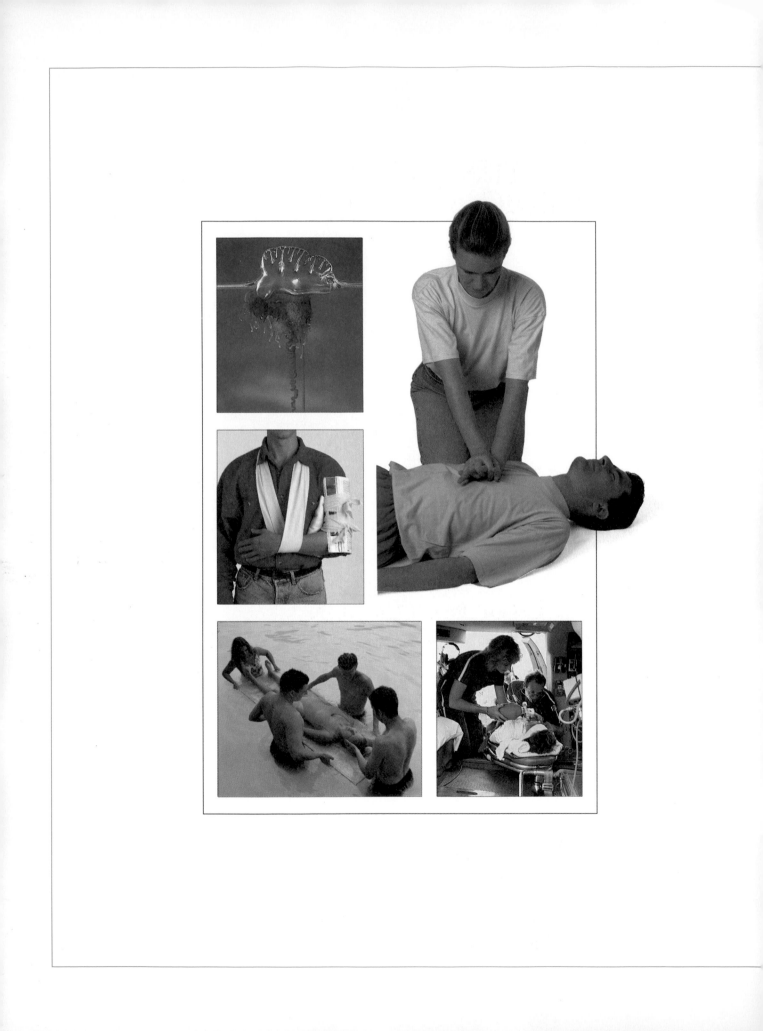

THE AMERICAN MEDICAL ASSOCIATION

ACCIDENTS AND EMERGENCIES

Medical Editor
CHARLES B. CLAYMAN, MD

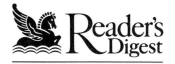

THE READER'S DIGEST ASSOCIATION, INC.
Pleasantville, New York/Montreal

The information in this book reflects current medical knowledge. The
recommendations and information are appropriate in most cases;
however, they are not a substitute for medical diagnosis. For specific
information concerning your personal medical condition, the AMA
suggests that you consult a physician.

The names of organizations, products, or alternative therapies appearing
in this book are given for informational purposes only. Their inclusion
does not imply AMA endorsement, nor does the omission of any
organization, product, or alternative therapy indicate AMA disapproval.

The AMA Home Medical Library is distinct from and unrelated to the
series of health books published by Random House, Inc., in conjunction
with the American Medical Association under the names "The AMA Home
Reference Library" and "The AMA Home Health Library."

Library of Congress Cataloging in Publication Data

Accidents and emergencies / medical editor, Charles B. Clayman.
     p.   cm.
    At head of title: The American Medical Association.
    Includes index.
    ISBN 0-89577-423-2
    1. Emergency medicine—Popular works. 2. First aid in illness and
injury—Popular works. I. Clayman, Charles B. II. American
Medical Association.
RC87.A32   1992
616.02'5—dc20   91-45392

FOREWORD

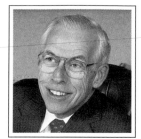

Accidental injury is the fourth leading cause of death among people of all ages. Children are at particularly high risk of accidental injury. Each year, one in every four children is injured seriously enough to need medical treatment. Young adults are at especially high risk of injuries caused by motor-vehicle accidents, while older people are more likely to be injured as a result of falls at home. Every year, accidental injuries take a terrible toll in terms of pain, disability, and death. They also cost billions of dollars in medical expenses and lost work time.

Many accidental injuries could be predicted and prevented. You and members of your family can take some simple safety steps to reduce your risk of accidental injury or even death. Think "safety" – whether you are at home, work, or enjoying your favorite leisure-time activity. Teach your children to recognize possible hazards and to make safety a habit.

This volume of the AMA Home Medical Library provides safety tips for home, work, and recreation. We include information every family needs to recognize the cause and type of injury or medical emergency and to give the appropriate first aid. We also explain how care is provided by the emergency medical services system – from emergency medical technicians at the scene to the hospital emergency department.

Unfortunately, preventive measures cannot guarantee safety, so it is extremely important that you learn the appropriate first-aid treatment in the event of an emergency. Action taken in the first few hours after an accident is critical – it may make the difference between life and death. We hope this volume provides helpful safety tips for you and members of your family and helps prepare you to act quickly if an accidental injury or medical emergency occurs.

James S. Todd MD

JAMES S. TODD, MD
Executive Vice President
American Medical Association

CONTENTS

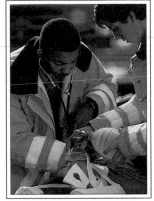

CHAPTER ONE

A SAFER LIFE-STYLE

STATISTICS SHOW that accidents and injuries can happen anytime and anywhere – at home, at work, during recreational activities, or in your car. Each year, almost 1 million people in the US are taken to a hospital emergency department as the result of a fall on stairs. Motor-vehicle accidents are the largest single cause of fatal injuries. However, in recent years, the number of deaths caused by motor-vehicle accidents has fallen as a result of measures such as improved safety design of vehicles, child safety seat laws, legislation to crack down on drinking and driving, 55-mile-per-hour speed limits on most highways, and the use of seat belts. Although some types of accidents may be unavoidable, in many cases preventive measures can greatly reduce the chances of you or someone you know being injured. Each of us can make our home safer by adopting some common-sense safety procedures and making these procedures part of our everyday routine. Unplugging small electrical appliances when they are not being used and locking up medications and household chemicals reduces the risk of fire and the likelihood of children accidentally poisoning themselves. If you have children, it is especially important that your home be safe because youngsters cannot always rec-

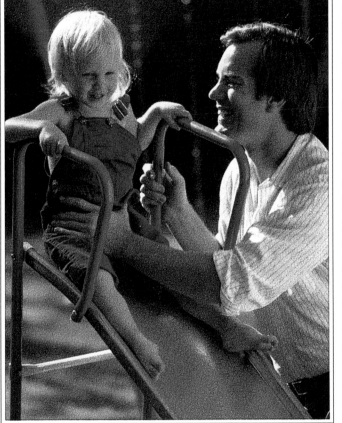

ognize and understand the hazards around them. Whatever activity you undertake, your risk of injury can be reduced by using tools or recreational equipment correctly. If you participate in sports, wearing the right clothing – including the correct shoes – can substantially reduce your risk of injury. When working in your garden or doing repairs at home, make sure you have the appropriate tools for the job and that you use them properly. Preventive safety measures are also very important in the workplace. Some occupations carry more risk than others. In the US, the probability of many types of injuries in the workplace has been reduced as a result of the Occupational Safety and Health Act. Employers must ensure that work conditions meet the safety standards established by this legislation. Employees are essential participants in a company's safety program. Safety regulations are effective only if you take responsibility for wearing all recommended protective clothing such as hard hats and safety goggles, are alert to potential hazards such as blocked emergency exits, and recommend change if your company's safety measures can be improved. This chapter gives safety recommendations for home, work, and recreation to help you reduce your risk of injury.

ACCIDENTS AND INJURIES

Of course, accidents are unexpected, and the toll they take in injury and death is terrible. But the term "accident" often describes a sequence of events that could have been prevented. Accidental injury is the fourth leading cause of death among people of all ages, accounting for about one in 20 deaths. The three most frequent causes of accidental death are motor-vehicle accidents, falls, and drownings. During the 1980s, more progress was made in reducing the total number of accidental deaths than in any previous decade. Accidental deaths were reduced by 10 percent, from 105,312 in 1979 to an estimated 94,500 in 1989.

CHILDREN AND YOUNG ADULTS

Accidents account for almost half of all deaths of children and young adults aged 1 to 24. In this broad age-group, motor-vehicle accidents are the leading cause of accidental death, killing about 16,000 people each year. Drownings are the next leading cause of death.

Among children under age 5, fires and drownings are the leading causes of accidental death. For infants under 1 year,

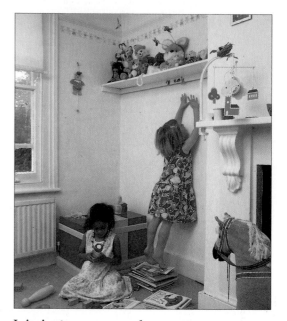

Injuries to young people
Young people are much more likely to be injured than adults. In young children, many injuries are the result of a fall or are associated with inappropriate or unsafe toys. In young adults, most injuries are caused by motor-vehicle accidents, followed by falls.

accidents account for about 3 percent of deaths and are the fifth leading cause of death. The incidence of accidental deaths rises sharply during the teenage years, with motor-vehicle accidents accounting for most of the increase.

Falls are by far the leading cause of accidental injury in infants. Among young children who fall, stairs, bicycles, roller skates, skateboards, and grocery store shopping carts are objects commonly associated with injuries.

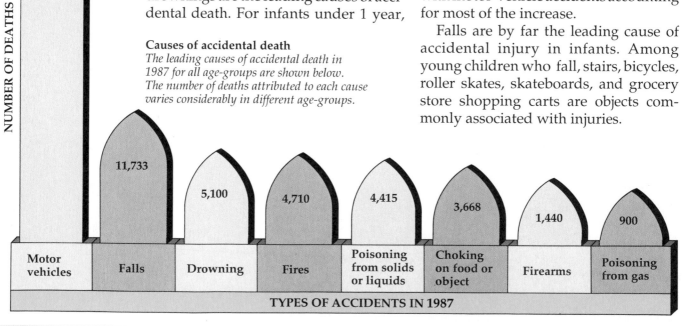

Causes of accidental death
The leading causes of accidental death in 1987 for all age-groups are shown below. The number of deaths attributed to each cause varies considerably in different age-groups.

NUMBER OF DEATHS

Motor vehicles	Falls	Drowning	Fires	Poisoning from solids or liquids	Choking on food or object	Firearms	Poisoning from gas
48,290	11,733	5,100	4,710	4,415	3,668	1,440	900

TYPES OF ACCIDENTS IN 1987

ACCIDENTS AND ALCOHOL OR OTHER DRUGS

Alcohol, illegal drugs of abuse, and some prescription drugs can impair judgment, reaction time, and muscle coordination. In 1988, about 50 percent of all traffic fatalities involved an intoxicated or alcohol-impaired driver or pedestrian. More than 8,100 sober drivers, passengers, and pedestrians died in alcohol-related accidents. Alcohol is also a factor in 29 percent of accidents resulting in serious injury and 7 percent of accidents resulting in property damage. About 300 deaths per year are attributed to poisoning from drinking a large amount of alcohol over a short period of time. The number of deaths caused by drug poisoning increased steadily in the 1980s – almost 4,000 such deaths occurred in 1987.

Ages of intoxicated drivers
The chart below shows the percentage of drivers with a blood alcohol concentration of 0.10 or greater (see page 36) in fatal crashes in 1988. The highest rates of alcohol intoxication were found in drivers in their early 20s.

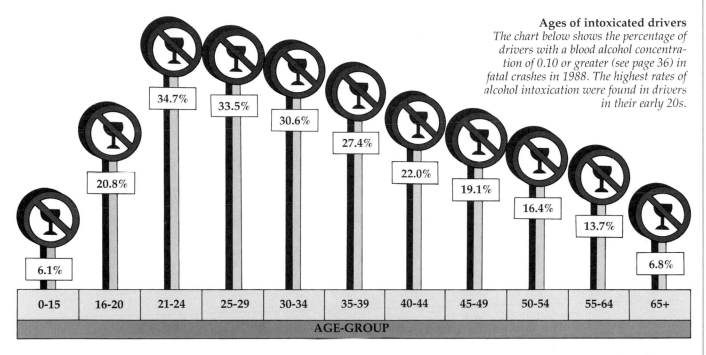

Age-group	Percentage
0-15	6.1%
16-20	20.8%
21-24	34.7%
25-29	33.5%
30-34	30.6%
35-39	27.4%
40-44	22.0%
45-49	19.1%
50-54	16.4%
55-64	13.7%
65+	6.8%

AGE-GROUP

ADULTS

Motor-vehicle accidents are the main cause of accidental death among people aged 25 to 44. Far more men die as the result of traffic accidents than women. The next leading cause of accidental death in this age-group is poisoning, followed by drownings, falls, and fires and burns. Common causes of nonfatal injuries in adults are falls, followed by motor-vehicle accidents, bumping into an object, and lifting and exertion.

OLDER PEOPLE

The fatal accidents that occur among older people vary by age-group. Up to age 79, motor-vehicle accidents are the most common cause of accidental death and falls are the second most common. This situation reverses after age 80. For people 90 and older, falls are the most common type of fatal accident, with suffocation by ingestion of food or other objects the second most common. Many of the accidents that occur among older people result from deteriorating health. For example, as a person's sense of balance and agility decline, the risk of falling becomes much greater. Many of the nonfatal injuries among older people are caused by falls, motor-vehicle accidents, burns, and poisoning.

Falls and older people
Bones become increasingly brittle as people age, making older people more likely to break bones during a fall than younger people. Each year, more than 200,000 older people fall and fracture their hips.

WHAT ARE THE HAZARDS AROUND US?

Accidental injury can lead to disability or death. For every accident that kills someone, there are 10 or more injuries that cause disability. But accident rates are headed in the right direction – downward. In 1989, death rates for motor-vehicle accidents and work-related accidents fell to all-time lows.

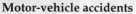

Motor-vehicle accidents
Motor-vehicle accidents are the leading cause of deaths and injuries. In 1989, 46,900 people, most of them between ages 15 and 24, were killed in motor-vehicle accidents. Two thirds of these deaths occurred in rural areas, and more than half occurred at night. Research has shown that, the higher the speed limit, the higher the rate of motor-vehicle accidents.

Sports injuries
Common sports injuries include fractures and strains and sprains of muscles, tendons, and ligaments. People injured during sports activities rarely die (except for swimmers or boaters who drown or rock climbers who fall). However, in 1988, six deaths occurred that were directly attributable to football injuries and 11 deaths were indirectly attributable to playing football (caused by vital-organ failure as a result of exertion or a complication).

Falls
Falls are the leading cause of accidental death in the home, accounting for about 6,000 deaths each year. Falls also cause many injuries (often fractures, bruises, and cuts and scrapes) that are treated in hospital emergency departments. Common causes of falls are slippery floors and icy or cracked, uneven sidewalks.

Poisoning
In 1989, 5,600 people died as a result of accidental poisoning. Over the last few decades, the death rate from accidental poisoning has more than doubled, from 0.8 to 1.8 per 100,000 people; the age-group 25 to 44 years had the greatest increase in death rate. The death rate for young children has fallen dramatically, mainly as a result of safer storage and disposal of household cleaning products and medications.

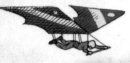

Violence

Intentional violent behavior – such as assault, rape, and homicide inside and outside the home – is a major cause of injury and death in the US. Appallingly, domestic violence is the single greatest cause of injury to women – women are more at risk in their homes than in their cars or on the streets. More than 2 million cases of child abuse are reported and 3 percent of the elderly are abused at home each year. Each year about 6 million people are victims of violent crime. Homicide and suicide are the leading causes of death in people aged 15 to 34. Intentional violence is an epidemic in our society.

Fires and burns

The number of people who die as a result of fires and burns has steadily declined in this century. In 1989, the death rate was 1.8 per 100,000 people (compared with 8.7 in 1920). In 1989, fires killed 4,400 people of all ages. In addition, burn injuries cause pain and suffering in many people every year. Fires started by cigarettes cause an estimated 1,500 deaths each year; many of the victims were infants, children, or disabled people.

Drowning

About 4,600 deaths were caused by drowning in 1989, making drowning the third leading cause of accidental death. About 2,800 people died while swimming or playing in water, and about 700 drownings were the result of boating accidents. Almost 25 percent of drowning victims were children; the majority of these children drowned in backyard swimming pools. Most of the remainder of drowning victims were young adults. Four times as many men as women drowned.

Environmental hazards

Extreme cold can cause frostbite and hypothermia; extreme heat can lead to heat exhaustion and heat stroke. Long-term sun exposure can lead to skin cancer. Other dangers include poisoning by toxic chemicals, hazardous waste, and various forms of radiation. Air pollution affects the air we breathe and the Earth's ozone layer, the destruction of which results in greater ultraviolet radiation from the sun.

SAFETY AT HOME

Increased awareness of home safety precautions has reduced the number of accidents in the home by 10 percent in the last 10 years. In 1988, one in 12 people needed medical attention for an injury that occurred at home. By identifying hazards and taking steps to help prevent accidents, you can reduce the risk of injury to you and your family.

ACCIDENTS IN THE HOME

Home accidents account for almost one fourth of all fatal injuries. The major factor that influences risk of injury is the age of the individual. Children under 5 have the highest rate of injury from home accidents, and people over 75 have

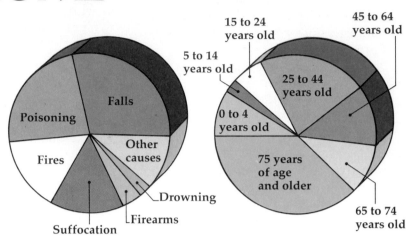

Fatal injuries in the home
In 1988, 22,500 fatal accidents occurred in the home. Falls, poisoning, fire-associated injuries, and suffocation from ingested objects were common causes of death.

Age distribution of fatal injuries in the home
People age 75 and over had more fatal injuries caused by accidents at home than any other age-group.

the greatest risk of being involved in a fatal accident at home. At all ages, males are at a slightly higher risk of accidental injury compared with females.

In the home, falls are the most common type of accident, followed closely by being struck by an object or getting cut. Nonfatal injuries in the home are usually cuts, bruises, bone fractures and dislocations, and burns, including scalds. Many types of minor injuries can be treated with a basic first-aid kit (see page 43). Make sure you check the supplies in your first-aid kit periodically to replace any used or outdated items. Store your first-aid kit in a place that is easily accessible in case of an emergency, yet out of the reach of infants and children.

MAKE A SAFETY CHECK

Some potential hazards in your home are obvious – such as your child's roller skates left lying at the top of the stairway. Other hazards may not be so easily identified, such as an extension cord that is beginning to crack. Your local library is a good source of information about

WHAT IS RADON?

Radon – a radioactive gas that is a product of the decay of uranium – has been claimed to be a cause of lung cancer among uranium miners. Radon may penetrate through cracks in the walls and foundation of a home, can contaminate the water, or can be emitted by some building materials. Good ventilation throughout your house reduces any possible risk. If you are concerned, call your public health department.

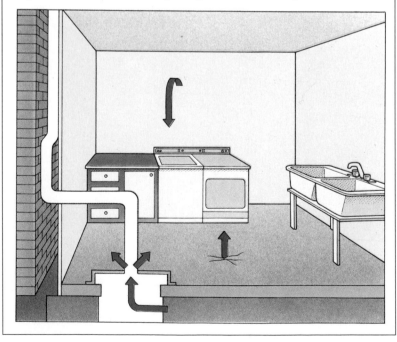

product safety and accident prevention in the home. You can also check with your local police or fire department or community center about safety programs that are available in your area.

On the basis of this information, inspect your home and the surrounding area and look for potential hazards. Make a list of dangers that you want to check for. You may want to make this type of safety check a regular family project to help reinforce the importance of accident prevention in your home. Make the necessary changes as soon as possible, starting with the hazards that pose the most serious risk.

Where are the dangers?

Accidents and injuries can occur in any part of your home. The cause is often a construction feature of a house, such as a staircase. Other household dangers include awkwardly placed furniture, slippery floors, loose rugs, and tools.

Hot liquids from pots and pans frequently cause scalds. Broken glass is a common cause of cuts. Sweep broken glass into a dustpan rather than using your hands to pick up the pieces. Wrap up broken glass and cans with sharp edges and put them in the garbage. Keep sharp items such as knives and nails out of the reach of children.

Accident statistics reveal some surprising hazards. If you have young children, never leave even a small amount of water or other liquid in a 5-gallon bucket. Your child can lean forward to reach into the bucket, then topple over and fall into the bucket headfirst. During the past 5 years, more than 100 toddlers have drowned in 5-gallon buckets.

Lead poisoning can pose a serious threat to children. Lead is present in some types of paint or in drinking water if your home has lead pipes, pipes connected with lead solder, or lead plumbing fixtures. Your local health department is a good source of information about testing the lead levels in your home.

DO-IT-YOURSELF SAFETY

No matter where you live, home and yard maintenance often involves using hand or power tools to make repairs. These tools can cause injury if they are used incorrectly, but taking a few safety precautions can minimize any risk. Read the manufacturer's instructions before using new equipment. Be sure to use the right tool for the type of repair job you are doing. Always replace damaged tools.

Eye protection
Don't take chances with your eyes. Always wear safety glasses or goggles when working with tools that might cause wood or metal particles or dust to enter your eyes.

Cutting tools
Keep the blades of your cutting tools sharp. You will need less physical effort to use the tools. Apply smooth, even pressure directed away from your body to cut, plane, or chisel. Always store tools out of reach of children after you use them.

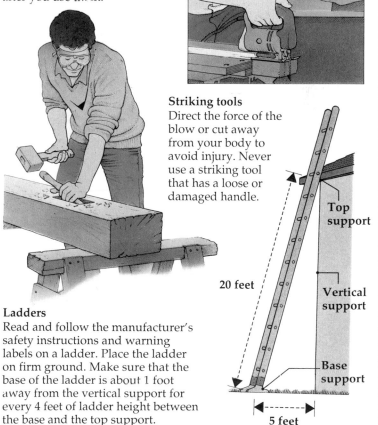

Striking tools
Direct the force of the blow or cut away from your body to avoid injury. Never use a striking tool that has a loose or damaged handle.

Top support

20 feet

Vertical support

Base support

5 feet

Ladders
Read and follow the manufacturer's safety instructions and warning labels on a ladder. Place the ladder on firm ground. Make sure that the base of the ladder is about 1 foot away from the vertical support for every 4 feet of ladder height between the base and the top support.

HOW TO PREVENT FIRES IN YOUR HOME

A small flame can grow into a fire that is burning out of control in just 30 seconds. Most fatalities in home fires occur between 10 PM and 6 AM, when most families are asleep. Few people are burned to death in fires; most people die from inhaling smoke and poisonous gases. Having smoke detectors and an emergency exit plan may save your family's life. You can help prevent fires by being aware of the common causes and by taking some simple safety precautions.

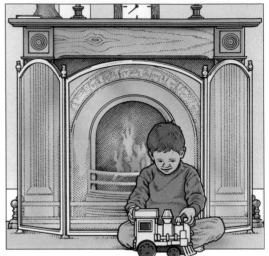

FIRE! HAVE AN EMERGENCY PLAN

You and your family should have periodic fire drills to practice the safest and quickest escape route. If fire strikes, remain calm and remember the following safety procedures:

◆ Call out to everybody in the house to alert them to the fire.
◆ Extinguish the fire only if you can do it without endangering life.
◆ If your clothes catch fire, don't run – stop, drop, and roll. Teach children this, too.
◆ If there is smoke in a room, crouch down below it and crawl to safety.
◆ If a door feels cool, open it a crack to check for smoke. If there is no smoke, follow your exit route, testing the warmth of all doors before you open them. Close the doors behind you as you go.
◆ Go directly to a predetermined meeting place outside your home.
◆ Use a neighbor's telephone to call the fire department.

Smoke detectors
Smoke detectors warn you of the presence of smoke. Put a smoke detector on every level of your home, including the basement. Be sure to put one near bedrooms. Test the batteries once a month and replace them at least once a year.

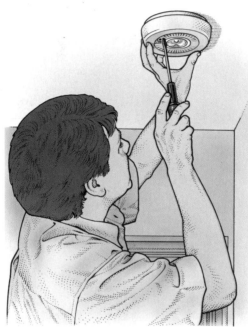

Electrical appliances
Make sure that any electrical appliance you buy has been safety-tested and approved. Read the owner's manual before using a new appliance. Make sure you are using fuses of the correct amperage for your appliances. Call an electrician if your appliances need checking.

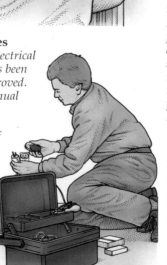

Children
Teach your child the dangers of playing with matches and lighters and keep them out of your child's reach. Never leave children alone where space heaters or stoves are being used. Keep fireplaces covered with screens or glass doors when using them.

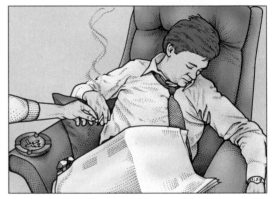

Smoking
In addition to the serious health hazards of smoking, fires attributable to smoking are the leading cause of deaths from fires in the home. The best health and safety advice is to quit smoking. If you are a smoker, never smoke if you are drowsy, are taking strong medication, or have drunk a large amount of alcohol – you may forget where you left a burning cigarette. Never, ever smoke in bed.

Flammable liquids
Store gasoline and other flammable liquids in safety containers in a workshed or the garage. Never pour flammable liquids near an open flame or light a cigarette near these liquids.

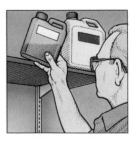

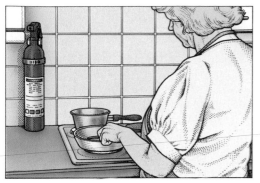

Older people

Older people should be particularly aware of the risk of fire. More than one third of all people who are injured or killed in a fire are over 65. About one third of the fire victims in this age-group started the fire that killed them, including fires caused by smoking and cooking.

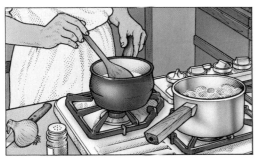

Stoves

Fires caused by stoves are the second largest cause of fires at home. When you are cooking, wear a short-sleeved shirt or roll up your sleeves to prevent your clothes from being ignited by the burners. Hang all pans, utensils, and spice racks away from your stove so that you do not have to reach across the stove to get them. Keep the broiler, ventilation ducts, and stove hoods free of grease.

Heating units
Heating units are the leading cause of fires and the second major cause of fire deaths. Have your furnace cleaned and checked once a year by a professional. Clean or change your furnace filters regularly to avoid overheating.

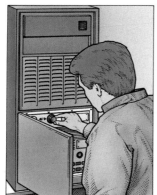

If you have a coal- or wood-burning heating system, make sure that the heating unit is at least 3 feet away from the wall and other objects and clean the stove, flue, and chimney once a year.

FIRE EXTINGUISHERS

Fire extinguishers are your first line of defense in case of small fires. Keep a fire extinguisher on each level of your home, including your basement. Read all the instructions on how to work the extinguisher. Check the extinguishers every month to make sure they are full and ready to use in case of a fire.

CLASS OF EXTINGUISHER	TYPE OF BURNING MATERIAL	CONTENTS OF EXTINGUISHER
A Class A	Wood, paper, cloth, cardboard, and most ordinary combustible materials	Water
B Class B	Flammable liquids such as oil, solvents, grease, and gases	Dry chemicals, carbon dioxide, or other substances that smother the fire
C Class C	Electrical equipment, such as electrical boxes and transformers	Dry chemicals, carbon dioxide, or other substances that smother the fire
D Class D	Combustible metals	Liquid or dry powder substance

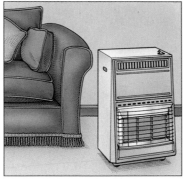

Space heaters
Be sure the room is well ventilated. Do not put a space heater close to furniture and position it so heat radiates into the room – not onto furniture. Portable heaters should be plugged directly into an outlet. If necessary, use a safety-approved, heavy-duty extension cord. Let the heater cool before you move it.

SAFE FUN ON THE FOURTH!

Celebrating the Fourth of July with fireworks is great fun but can be extremely dangerous to adults as well as children. Don't risk it! Leave the fireworks celebration to professionals – go to the fireworks display in your community. Every year, thousands of people (about half of whom are under 15 years old) are treated in hospital emergency departments for fireworks-related injuries. Fireworks – even sparklers – burn at very high temperatures and can easily set your clothing or home on fire.

A safe garage and yard
Tools used in the garden or for home repairs should always be put away after use, especially if they have sharp edges or points. Wearing gloves reduces the likelihood of infection – including tetanus – caused by bacteria or fungi in the soil.

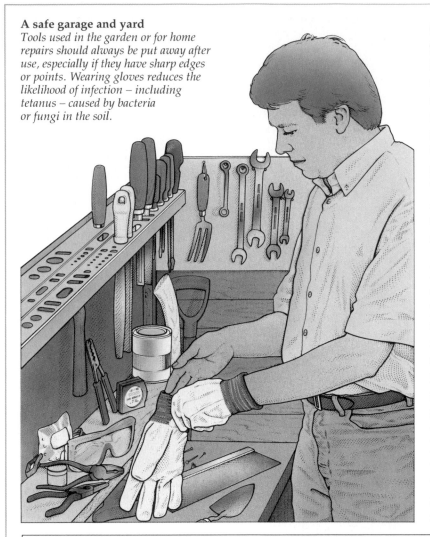

Outside your home

Safety precautions are also important to help prevent injuries when you are working in your garage or yard or your children are playing outside. Garden tools, especially rakes or sharp implements such as pruning shears or hedge trimmers, should never be left on the ground. Be sure to pick up nails to prevent someone from stepping on them. All gardening chemicals, paints, and cleaning agents should be sealed properly and kept out of reach of children.

Wearing gloves while gardening can help protect you against tetanus and other types of infection. Make sure that you and your family are up-to-date on tetanus shots. Children should be immunized at 2, 4, 6, and 18 months and at 4 to 6 years of age. Booster shots are usually needed every 5 to 10 years; a booster shot may be needed sooner if you have a severe wound. The spores of the bacteria that cause tetanus infection live in soil. Infection can result if these spores enter the body through a cut or puncture wound. About 100 cases of tetanus are reported every year, most occurring in nonimmunized people over 50.

FIREARM SAFETY

There are about 70 million firearm owners in the US who possess 200 million firearms. Some people believe that the best way to protect themselves is to own a firearm and that handgun ownership is a crime deterrent. In fact, firearms were used in almost three out of five homicides committed in the US. Furthermore, more than 1,400 people died in firearm-related accidents in 1990, and 800 of these accidents occurred at home. If you own a firearm, it is essential that you understand the potential dangers of having a gun in your home. Know how to use and handle the firearm properly, and keep it stored in a safe place.

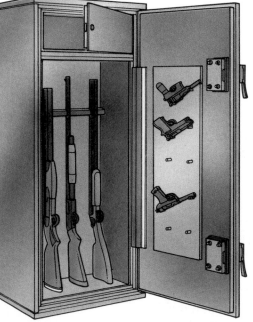

Safely storing firearms
If you own a firearm, store it unloaded and uncocked in a securely locked case. Keep your ammunition away from heat or moisture and in a separate location in a locked container. Childproof a revolver by placing a padlock around the top strap of the weapon (so that the cylinder cannot be flipped into position) or by using a trigger lock. One in 30 deaths of children in 1990 was firearm-related. Each year, accidental shootings in the home kill about 250 children 14 years old and younger.

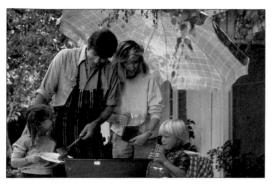

Barbecuing safely
Keep a close eye on children when you are barbecuing. Fire is fascinating to a curious child. Your child may be burned if he or she touches or brushes up against a hot grill. If your child plays too close to a hot grill, it may accidentally tip over and fall on the child. Never barbecue in an enclosed area.

Risks for older people

Older people are especially at risk of injury from falls. Falls among older people are often associated with failing eyesight, loss of the sense of balance, or difficulty walking. The side effects of some medications may also impair the person's perception of his or her surroundings. Climbing up or down a flight of stairs can become particularly hazardous for an older person; a handrail that extends along the entire length of the stairway reduces the risk of falling.

Uneven floors can trip anyone, especially someone who is unsteady on his or her feet. Replace slippery floor coverings and fasten frayed and loose carpet edges. Safe, comfortable shoes are important. Worn-down heels should be repaired and shoes with worn-out soles should be repaired or replaced. In the winter you can help prevent accidents by clearing snow from stairs and sidewalks, salting icy walks, and running errands for older relatives.

If you are concerned about the safety of an older relative or friend who lives alone, emergency alert devices are available. In an emergency, the wearer pushes a button on the device that automatically dials programmed numbers on the telephone to call for help from a neighbor, relative, or monitoring service.

IS YOUR ELECTRICAL WIRING SAFE?

Most people do not have the expertise to tackle electrical rewiring jobs in their homes. If you have any doubts about the safety of your wiring (for instance, if fuses blow regularly), have your wiring checked by an electrician. Electric shocks and fires can be prevented by following these rules.

One plug, one socket
Using too many adapters in a single socket can overload the wiring and cause an electrical fire. Multiple-plug extension bars are available that have a built-in safety shutoff if the electrical socket becomes overloaded. To pull the plug from the socket, grip the plug – not the cord.
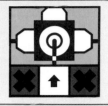

Water and electricity
Water conducts electricity. Never touch electrical switches or sockets if your hands are wet; dry your hands thoroughly first. Electrical appliances should never be used near a sink, tub, or toilet because they could fall in the water.
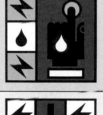

Cutoff switches
Electrical tools can short-circuit and give you a shock. Use an electrical outlet that has a ground-fault circuit interrupter, which is designed to cut off the power if it detects an electrical leak from the circuit. Power tools should be turned off and unplugged after use.
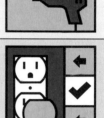

Electrical outlet covers
Infants and young children can be injured by electric shock from uncovered wall outlets. Covers for electrical outlets are available; these covers are inserted into the outlet and help prevent an infant or child from inserting small objects into the outlet.
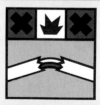

Damaged or worn electrical cords
A damaged or worn electrical cord should never be temporarily repaired with tape; replace it to prevent fire and electrical shock. Burns in and around the mouth occur to children who bite through damaged or even intact electrical cords.
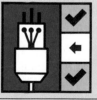

Wiring a plug
When rewiring an electric plug, be sure that the wiring is connected to the correct terminals on the plug, that there are no loose connections, and that the wiring's protective covering is stripped down no farther than is necessary to make the connections inside the plug.

Extension cords
Use extension cords carefully. Hidden under a carpet, an extension cord may overheat and cause a fire. Securing extension cords to walls with approved clips prevents fires and ensures that your family will not trip over the cords.
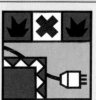

PROTECTING CHILDREN FROM INJURY

The most common types of injuries among children differ according to age-groups. In children under 4, a 1-year-old baby is the most prone to falls, cuts, and burns. Accidents involving a curious, unsupervised 2-year-old child often include poisoning by swallowing medications or household cleaning products. At 4 years, bone fractures from falls are a common injury. Fatal injuries are twice as likely to occur among boys than girls. The number of children who are injured as a result of preventable accidents, particularly injuries caused by falling out of windows, increases dramatically during the warm-weather months.

Children need constant supervision. Never leave an infant or preschool-age child alone. Make sure any preteen or teen you hire as a babysitter is mature enough to handle the responsibility. Even children who are supervised can have accidents; it takes only a moment for a mishap to occur.

Car trips
All children who weigh 40 pounds or less (some experts suggest 60 pounds or less) must sit in a child's car seat that is appropriate for the child's height and weight. The seat should be secured with the vehicle's safety belt in the center of the back seat. For children who weigh less than 20 pounds, the recommended position for the car seat is with the infant and seat facing the back of the car.

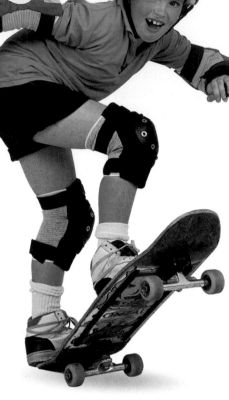

Children at play
Seven out of 10 playground injuries are caused by falls. Make sure the layout and construction of your child's playground and the equipment are safe, and teach your child the rules of safe play (see page 35). If your child enjoys skateboarding or roller skating, make sure he or she wears protective clothing (a helmet and elbow and knee pads) and stays off the street.

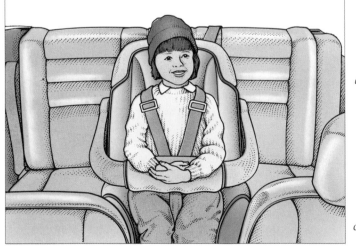

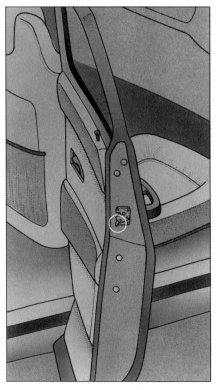

Childproof locks
Childproof locks on rear doors are available on some car models. These locks have a latch in the side panel of the doors that can be engaged to prevent the rear doors from being opened from the inside. Window locks prevent a child from lowering or changing the position of the car windows.

POISONOUS SUBSTANCES IN YOUR HOME

Poisoning can result from swallowing toxic solids or liquids or from inhaling harmful fumes. Inquisitive children can easily poison themselves with household products, especially those that do not taste bad – such as ant killers, roach powders, and furniture polish. All potentially harmful substances should be kept in a locked cabinet or in a cabinet out of your children's reach. If you store household products under the kitchen sink, install childproof latches. If your child is poisoned, call your local poison control center for first-aid instructions. Write down the name of the substance or bring the container and/or the substance with you to the emergency department.

HOUSEHOLD PRODUCTS

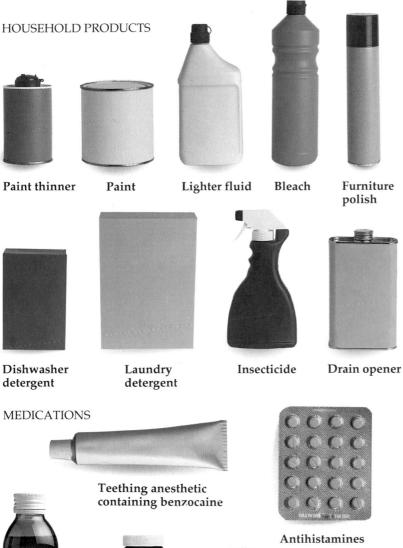

| Paint thinner | Paint | Lighter fluid | Bleach | Furniture polish |

| Dishwasher detergent | Laundry detergent | Insecticide | Drain opener |

MEDICATIONS

Teething anesthetic containing benzocaine

Antihistamines

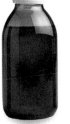

| Cough medicine | Vitamins | Aspirin or acetaminophen | Prescription medicine |

Q My pharmacist always puts my medication in containers that have childproof safety caps. How "childproof" are these containers?

A Childproof containers could be more accurately called child-resistant containers. Although a young child may be able to remove the safety cap, it is much more difficult to take off than a regular lid. Make sure you replace the safety cap properly and always keep all medications out of the reach of your children.

Q The water in our bathroom is very hot and I am afraid that one of my children will get scalded. What can I do to prevent this?

A To prevent scalding, adjust your water heater temperature to 120 to 130 degrees or install antiscald devices on your faucets. Scalding is a serious danger for children. Always stay with your children when they are bathing or showering. Unsupervised toddlers may fall into bathwater and be unable to get out, or they may turn a hot water handle. Teach your children to test the water before getting into a bathtub.

Q I have done a safety check of my home and think that I have put everything potentially harmful out of my children's reach. What more can I do?

A Teach your children about the potential dangers around them. Many communities have programs to help teach your child about home safety. Make sure your child knows how to call 911 (or the emergency number in your area) in case of an emergency and is able to give his or her full name and address.

IS YOUR HOME CHILDPROOF?

Children have more accidents and injuries than adults. Many of these injuries can be prevented simply by making a child's environment a safer place to play in and explore. A home that is safe for your child will also be a safer place for you.

BATHROOM
Lock up all medications or store them in a cabinet that is out of your child's reach.

Keep the lids on toilet seats down.

Install safety glass in shower doors or use shower curtains.

Radiators should not be too hot to touch. If necessary, turn down the thermostat or install radiator covers.

Install grab rails at the edge of the bathtub. Use nonskid mats or adhesive safety strips in the tub.

SWIMMING POOL AND YARD
Never leave a child alone near a pool; a child can drown in a pool that contains only 2 inches of water. Do not use flotation devices as a substitute for your constant supervision.

Completely remove a pool cover. Children can become trapped under a partially removed cover.

Keep rescue equipment and a telephone near the pool.

Remove steps from an above-ground pool when it is not in use.

Put a climb-proof fence around your yard or pool. The fence should have a self-closing gate, with the latch out of reach of children.

Surround play equipment with soft ground, such as grass, sand, or pea-sized gravel.

Always put gardening and other tools away after use.

Make sure the plants in your garden are not poisonous.

GARAGE
Store tools in locked toolboxes. Lock away all chemicals.

Lock freezers or refrigerators.

Make sure your electric garage door opener has a safety system that stops and reverses the door when it touches an object in its path.

Keep all 5-gallon buckets completely empty.

KITCHEN
Use the back burners on the stove. Turn pot and pan handles toward the back.

Install antiscald devices on faucets or set your water heater at 120 to 130 degrees.

Unplug all small appliances when you are not using them.

Keep matches, sharp items, and household cleaners in a locked cabinet or out of reach of children. Install safety latches on cabinets at child-level.

Keep a fire extinguisher and first-aid kit in the kitchen.

CHILD'S BEDROOM
Use flame-resistant bedding and make sure your child has flame-resistant pajamas.

Use outlet covers on unused electrical outlets in the house.

Install safety locks on all windows in the house so that children cannot open them more than 2 inches.

Do not let a baby under 1 year old use pillows; the baby may suffocate.

Children's furniture should be low, soft, and have no sharp edges. A toy chest should also have a lightweight lid that does not latch.

Put only a few small, soft toys in the crib. Lower the level of the mattress as your child grows and learns to stand in the crib. A child can use large toys as "stepping-stones" to climb out of the crib.

Any vertical bars on a child's bed or crib should be no more than 2 inches apart. Mechanisms that lower the side of the crib should lock automatically when the side is returned to the raised position.

STAIRS
Make sure that handrails extend the entire length of stairways. Keep stairways well lit and remove loose or worn carpeting. Use nonslip area rugs or throw rugs on floors at the top and bottom of stairways.

Use safety gates at the top and bottom of the stairs. Keep the stairs clear of clutter.

Install a smoke detector on each level of your home and above the foot of the stairs where smoke gathers as it rises up the stairway. Check the batteries in your smoke detectors monthly and replace them immediately when necessary.

Place a screen or install glass doors over fireplaces.

Keep potted plants out of reach. Pots within reach could topple down on your child's head. Make sure that your household plants are not poisonous.

Keep floors clear of tripping hazards.

All chairs and sofas should be made of flame-resistant materials.

LIVING ROOM
Position the television so that your child cannot reach the back of the set.

Taking precautions

In 1988, about 4,700 children died from swallowing poisonous household substances. Some products, such as drain cleaners, are so caustic (corrosive) that, if swallowed, they can cause permanent damage to a child's mouth and throat. To protect your child, follow the safety precautions given on page 21.

Put away in a safe place small items that could be swallowed or cause choking. Small items that a school-age child can safely play with may pose a great danger to a younger brother or sister if left within reach. Plastic bags should always be kept out of reach of children to prevent the possibility of suffocation.

Safety guidelines for all types of nursery equipment and toys can be obtained at your local library or by calling the Consumer Product Safety Commission (800-638-2772). Before buying an item, check the safety guidelines for that item and ask the salesperson for a demonstration of safety features.

Safety gates
Safety gates should be installed on stairways to prevent children from falling. Safety gates should be securely fitted to the top and bottom of the staircase. Gates with a straight top edge and rigid mesh screen are recommended. Toddlers learning to crawl or walk up stairs should be supervised closely. Toddlers are especially at risk if they are carrying toys or other items, because they cannot hold onto railings or walls.

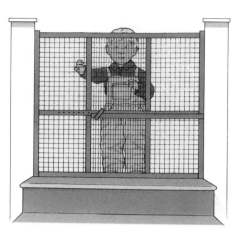

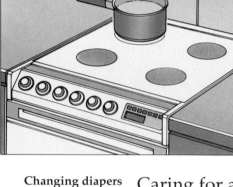

Scalds
Teach your child not to touch the stove. Keep hot liquids out of his or her reach (see pages 22 and 25). Never carry boiling water or other hot liquids around small children. Even a slight spill could cause a severe scald.

Changing diapers
A baby can wiggle and roll amazingly quickly. Before putting your baby on a changing table or bed, have all items you need within reach; keep one hand on your baby at all times.

Caring for an injured child

If your child has an accident, give the appropriate first aid for the injury (see TYPES OF INJURIES on pages 60 to 121). In cases of serious injuries, call 911 (or the emergency number in your community) or take the child to the nearest hospital emergency department. If possible, tell a neighbor where you are going, make sure electrical appliances are turned off, and lock up the house.

The doctor will need to know how your child's injury happened. His or her questions are not intended to be judgmental or critical. For example, if the injury is a scald, the doctor will want to know what the liquid was, how long the liquid was boiled or was heated, what the child was wearing over the scalded area, and whether you cooled the scalded area immediately. All of these questions help to determine the appropriate treatment based on the doctor's evaluation of how badly the skin has been burned.

CASE HISTORY
A PREVENTABLE ACCIDENT

M ANDY WAS PLAYING with her dolls in the kitchen while her mother, Jill, prepared their lunch. The doorbell rang and Jill went to answer the door. It was her neighbor and close friend, Carol. While her mother was away, Mandy decided to help with lunch by checking to see if the hot dogs that were boiling on the stove were ready to eat. Jill and Carol heard Mandy scream and ran into the kitchen.

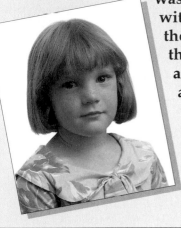

PERSONAL DETAILS
Name Mandy Lawrence
Age 5
Occupation Kindergarten student
Family Mandy is an only child.

THE INCIDENT

Jill and Carol find Mandy sitting on the floor in front of the stove screaming in pain and clutching her arm. The pot that her mother has been using to boil the hot dogs is overturned on the floor. Jill realizes that Mandy must have reached up to the stove and tipped the pot over, spilling the boiling water onto her arm. Carol turns off the stove while Jill tries to soothe her frightened child.

FIRST AID

Jill asks Carol to get some butter out of the refrigerator to put on Mandy's arm. Carol tells Jill that you should never put anything but cold water from the faucet on a burn, letting the water run on the burn for at least 5 minutes. After running cold water on the burn, Carol helps Jill wrap the burn in clean gauze and then drives Mandy and Jill to the hospital emergency department.

AT THE HOSPITAL

When they arrive at the hospital, Jill tells the doctor how Mandy's arm got burned. The nurse wets the gauze with cold water as the doctor unwraps Mandy's arm. Most of the upper part of her arm has been scalded and blisters have formed. The doctor gives Mandy a pain medication. He cleans the burn, applies an antibacterial cream to prevent infection, and covers the burn with a sterile gauze dressing. The doctor tells Jill to change the dressing two to three times a day and to make an appointment with Mandy's pediatrician for a follow-up examination within the next 2 days. The doctor tells Jill that she did the right thing by running cold water over the burn. He explains that putting ointments or butter on a burn makes it harder to clean and may cause infection. The doctor then asks Jill a few additional questions about how the accident happened. He explains to her that he is required by law to investigate the injury to rule out the possibility of child abuse. Jill says she understands completely, answers all his questions, and says she will never again leave Mandy alone in the kitchen with boiling water on the stove.

THE OUTCOME

Two days later, Mandy's pediatrician examines the burn and tells Jill that Mandy's arm will heal but there may be a slight scar. The doctor then advises Jill on how to prevent such accidents in the future. Jill learns that she should use the back burners on the stove and turn the handles of pans toward the back of the stove, out of Mandy's reach.

Treating the burn
In the emergency department, the doctor checks the severity of the burn. He cleans the burned area, applies an antibacterial cream to prevent infection, and wraps Mandy's arm in a sterile dressing.

SAFETY AT WORK

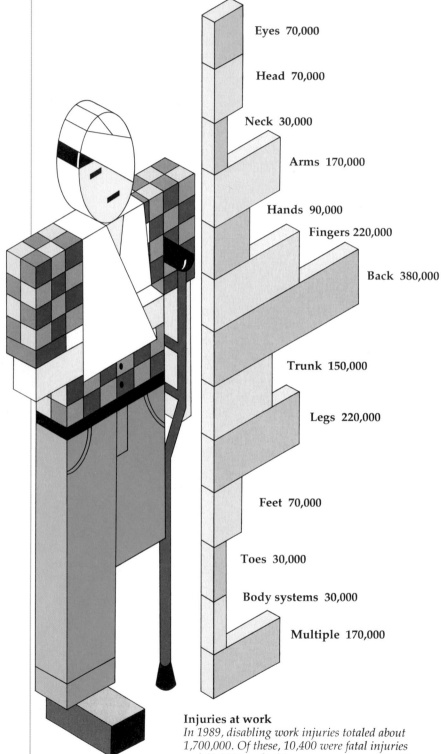

Eyes 70,000

Head 70,000

Neck 30,000

Arms 170,000

Hands 90,000

Fingers 220,000

Back 380,000

Trunk 150,000

Legs 220,000

Feet 70,000

Toes 30,000

Body systems 30,000

Multiple 170,000

Injuries at work
In 1989, disabling work injuries totaled about 1,700,000. Of these, 10,400 were fatal injuries and 60,000 resulted in some permanent disability. The chart above shows the parts of the body most frequently injured at work. Injuries to the back occur most frequently, followed by thumb and finger injuries and leg injuries.

The Occupational Safety and Health Act (OSHA) was passed by Congress in 1970 to help ensure safe and healthy working conditions. This act sets the standards, rules, and regulations by which employers are required to protect their employees on the job. Even though your employer has a responsibility to protect you and your fellow employees, you can also play an active role in reducing the risk of injury in your workplace.

WORK-RELATED INJURIES

Many injuries at work are a result of improper physical conditioning and mismatches between a person's physical capabilities and the demands of the task. Injuries are also frequently caused by slips and falls and by striking or being struck by an object. In 1989, 35 million work days were lost as a result of work-related injuries. Between 1912 and 1989, the number of deaths caused by work-related injuries decreased by 81 percent—from 21 to four deaths per 100,000 people each year. In 1912 about 20,000 people died in the workplace. In 1989, with a total work force more than three times as large, 10,400 people died.

Reducing your risk

How can you help protect yourself from injury at work? Companies with excellent safety records always cite cooperative employees as essential to a successful injury prevention program. Consider how you perform the tasks of your job and the conditions in your workplace that may be hazardous to your health. Become thoroughly familiar with safety procedures and protective equipment. Examine the equipment that you work with and learn about injuries commonly associated with your occupation, craft, or profession. A better understanding of the potential dangers will help you protect yourself and your coworkers against injury. Take time to follow safety procedures and encourage your coworkers to do the same. Some health risks are recognized only after injuries or illnesses have been reported, so it is important to report any such occurrence to your supervisor or manager.

If you are seeking employment, consider your potential employer's safety record. If you are concerned about safety in your workplace, talk to your supervisor or manager about your concerns. You can offer to become involved in a safety program or committee. If you have repeatedly reported a hazard and no corrective action is taken by your employer, contact the Occupational Safety and Health Administration's local office and file a written complaint.

IDENTIFYING POTENTIAL HAZARDS

The types of hazards in the workplace and the risk of injury vary among different occupations. Find out about any occupational health-risk factors that may be present at your company. Make sure you know the location of your workplace's first-aid station. All equipment is potentially dangerous if used incorrectly. Make sure that you understand how to work all equipment that you come in contact with and check the safety features on the equipment.

Determining the types of energy that are generated at your workplace is important in preventing injury. Heat can cause burns, laser beams may damage your eyes, loud tools or machinery may impair your hearing, electricity can cause electrocution or burns, and strong air or water pressure from hoses can cause skin damage and internal injury. To prevent such injuries, make sure that the machinery you use has the appropriate safety features and that you wear the recommended safety clothing.

PERSONAL PROTECTION – HEAD TO TOE

Many industries are required by law to provide appropriate personal protective equipment or clothing for their employees. Such equipment can protect you from injury only if you wear it routinely, it fits well, and it fully covers the area of your body that is exposed to injury.

Ears
Do you need earplugs or other devices to protect against high levels of noise?

Nose
Do you need a mask to keep you from inhaling dust or chemicals? If you work with harmful fumes, is there an adequate ventilator on the mask? Is the mask suited to the type of chemicals you are exposed to?

Limbs
Can moving machinery cut, crush, or entangle your fingers, hands, arms, legs, or feet? If so, remove rings, watches, and bracelets to prevent them from being caught in moving machinery and wear protective clothing.

Feet
Are your feet at risk of injury from machinery or falling objects? If so, wear appropriate safety shoes. Wear shoes with reinforced soles to prevent cuts and punctures and shoes with safety toes to protect your feet from falling objects.

Head
Do you need to wear a form of head protection, such as a hard hat?

Eyes
Do you need to protect your eyes? If so, wear safety goggles. Make sure that lighting is sufficient to prevent straining your eyes.

Mouth
Can contaminants enter your mouth by splashing in your face or on your fingers? Are washing facilities adequate?

Back
If you lift heavy objects, use the correct technique (see page 28) and keep the muscles of your back and abdomen well-toned and strong.

Skin
Do you need protective clothing or gloves to safeguard your skin against abrasion, friction, heat, cold, or exposure to hazardous chemicals?

EMERGENCY PROCEDURES AND SAFETY MANUALS

Instructions for emergency procedures in the event of fire or power outages should be available from your employer or building management office. Some companies provide employees with a safety manual. If safety instructions are not available, you should suggest to your supervisor or manager that they be prepared. The information in company safety manuals is in your best interest, and both employers and employees must follow the guidelines to ensure the safest possible working environment.

Fire in the workplace

Your company's safety procedures should tell you what to do in the event of a fire. Be sure you know the location of fire extinguishers and fire exits. If a fire starts, call the fire department. Attempt to put out a fire only if it does not endanger the safety of you or your coworkers. If you must evacuate the building, go to the nearest fire exit. Use designated stairways only – never use an elevator.

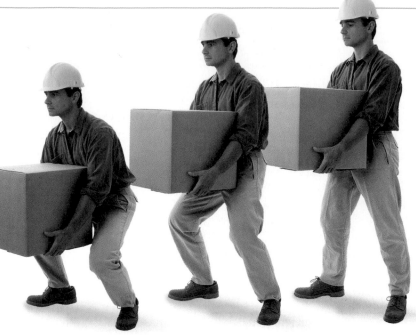

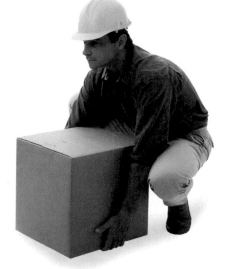

Lifting carefully
If your job requires you to do a lot of lifting, make sure that your footing is stable, your back is straight and almost upright, and your body is centered over your feet. Get a good grasp on the object and pull it close to you; lift with your legs – not your back. Move your feet to turn; do not twist your back.

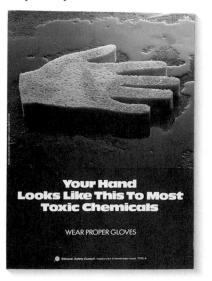

Pay attention!
Reading and heeding posted safety procedures and warnings, as well as other forms of safety information from your employer, could prevent an injury or even save your life.

Preventing personal injury

You can reduce the risk of some types of injury by making sensible choices about your work habits and environment. To help prevent backstrain, sit straight at your desk and adjust your chair if necessary to provide support for the lower part of your back. Use proper techniques when you lift objects to avoid straining your back muscles (see above). Make sure you have appropriate and comfortable footwear. Keep yourself physically fit for your work, and stay alert on the job. If you experience recurrent pain that you think might be related to your work, talk to your doctor.

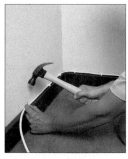

Preventing falls
You can reduce your risk of falling or tripping by keeping your work space clear of spilled liquids or objects such as electrical cords and waste.

SPECIFIC HAZARDS

Some occupations carry specific health and safety risks, such as working with chemicals, dusts, volatile and flammable vapors, radiation and lasers, or sharp instruments or equipment. Your occupation may require that you work at a great height, in a confined space, or even under water. These risk factors require that you take specific safety precautions. The best way to avoid injury is to find out as much as you can about your particular type of work and make sure that you follow all safety instructions carefully.

Chemical burns

Chemical burns are a frequent form of serious injury. If you work with chemicals, check your company safety manual or ask your supervisor for written instructions on safe work practices for handling these substances. In a study conducted in 1985, two thirds of workers who were injured by chemical burns said they had worn some type of personal protective equipment, most often gloves, boots, and goggles. But only one third reported that their equipment was resistant to the chemicals and three fourths said that their protective clothing did not cover the burn area. Of the injured workers, one third said that they did not think protection was necessary. In some cases, workers were burned despite wearing chemical-resistant clothing. In most cases, burns occurred because the clothing was in poor condition, did not fit properly, or was the wrong type to protect against the chemical being used. Many injuries can be prevented by regular review and monitoring of safety procedures, regular use of appropriate protective clothing, and compliance with established safety guidelines.

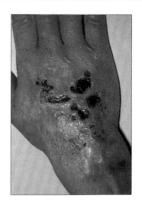

Injuries from chemicals
Every year many workers are injured as a result of chemical burns, even though the injured employees are familiar with the chemicals. The burns shown above were caused by lime, a corrosive chemical widely used in the construction industry.

REPETITIVE STRAIN INJURY

Repeating the same movement during your workday can cause strain, discomfort, and disability. These problems are called repetitive strain injury or cumulative trauma – a condition that develops over time and affects muscles, bones, or nerves. The most commonly affected areas are the wrists, hands, and fingers. To reduce your risk of repetitive strain injury, use the proper tool for the job, minimize the speed and force of the repeated movement, change the design of your workstation to maintain a comfortable working posture, and take periodic breaks, if possible.

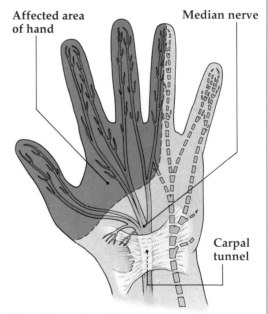

Affected area of hand **Median nerve**

Carpal tunnel

Trigger finger
Trigger finger is sometimes caused by the repeated flexing of a finger under pressure, such as occurs when using trigger-operated hand tools. Symptoms are pain, swelling, tenderness, and weakness in the affected fingers and hands. Treatment involves avoiding tasks that require repeated flexing of the affected finger, resting the hand, and taking anti-inflammatory drugs.

Carpal tunnel syndrome
Carpal tunnel syndrome is the result of compression of the median nerve (above). It can be caused by repeatedly flexing and extending the wrist. Symptoms are pain, numbness, tingling, burning, and weakness in the hand and fingers. Treatment involves resting the wrist and taking anti-inflammatory drugs. Sometimes injections of a corticosteroid drug or surgery is required.

SAFETY IN RECREATION

In recent years, people in the US have become more health conscious than ever before and have a greater awareness of the importance of staying physically fit. As a result, more people are participating in sports and other forms of exercise. The physical benefits of regular exercise include improved mobility, stronger muscles, greater stamina, and a reduced risk of heart disease and degenerative bone disorders such as osteoporosis. Recreation also helps people relax, which can prevent and alleviate the adverse effects of stress. But participating in sports and other recreational activities also increases your potential for injury. Before beginning a new activity that involves physical exertion, make sure it is appropriate for your current level of physical fitness. Your doctor can help you decide. For many sports it is vital that you receive training and instruction and that you use the correct equipment and protective clothing.

EVALUATING YOUR FITNESS LEVEL

Age is never a barrier to staying in shape. However, if you are over 40, talk to your doctor before you start a new physical activity, especially if you have a family history of high blood pressure or heart disease. If you are recovering from an injury or illness, or if you have general symptoms such as weakness or tiredness, consult your doctor before participating in any strenuous activity.

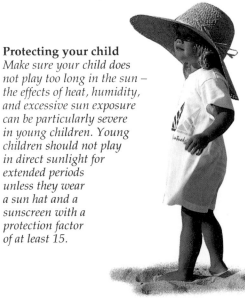

Clothing for cold weather
In cold weather, it is important to dress correctly. Several layers of cotton clothing provide better insulation than one thick layer. Layers also allow you to remove clothes as you heat up during your workout. At least 20 percent of body heat is lost through your head – in cold weather, wear a warm hat that covers your ears.

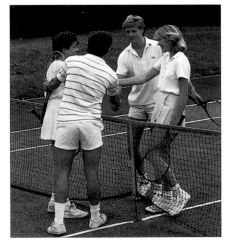

Take it slow and easy
When you begin a new exercise or sport, build up your level of fitness gradually to reduce your risk of injury. Many sports injuries result from trying to do too much too soon.

Protecting your child
Make sure your child does not play too long in the sun – the effects of heat, humidity, and excessive sun exposure can be particularly severe in young children. Young children should not play in direct sunlight for extended periods unless they wear a sun hat and a sunscreen with a protection factor of at least 15.

PREVENTING INJURY

The injury rate among professional athletes is relatively low because their physical fitness level is high and they train intensively. Many people participating in recreational sports push themselves too hard and too fast without any physical conditioning; injuries occur as a result of this overexertion.

The best way to prevent injury in any sport is to maintain a constant level of physical fitness through exercise that is not overly stressful. Perform a regular exercise routine several times a week rather than being a "weekend warrior," exercising only occasionally, too strenuously, and overexerting yourself. Eat a well-balanced diet that provides you with sufficient calories as well as the vitamins and minerals you need to keep up with your energy expenditure.

If you do get hurt, be sure you allow yourself enough time to recover. Returning to sports activities too quickly can cause reinjury, sometimes resulting in more severe damage to the injured area.

Participating in any exercise activity is dangerous if you have been drinking alcohol or taking medication that makes you feel drowsy. Alcohol and some other drugs can cause lapses in concentration and loss of coordination, both of which increase your chances of injury.

Second injury syndrome
Second injury syndrome occurs when a minor injury is followed by a second injury. A second injury may occur as a result of trying to protect an already injured, painful part of your body. This type of injury is more common in a person who does not participate in an activity regularly.

WARM-UP AND COOL-DOWN EXERCISES

Before any form of exercise, give yourself a warm-up to prepare your body for the increased level of exertion. A warm-up routine should include stretching exercises, which reduce the risk of injury by increasing your flexibility. After your exercise routine or strenuous physical activity, cool down by repeating the stretching exercises (see below).

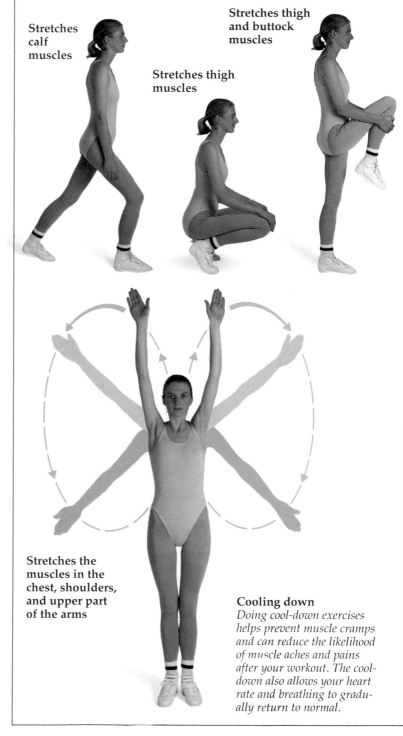

Stretches calf muscles

Stretches thigh muscles

Stretches thigh and buttock muscles

Stretches the muscles in the chest, shoulders, and upper part of the arms

Cooling down
Doing cool-down exercises helps prevent muscle cramps and can reduce the likelihood of muscle aches and pains after your workout. The cool-down also allows your heart rate and breathing to gradually return to normal.

HOW TO ENJOY WATER ACTIVITIES SAFELY

Many people enjoy activities that take place both in and around water. All water sports can be dangerous, even if you are a good swimmer; drownings are the third leading cause of accidental death. When you are around water you should always be with at least one other person in case someone is injured or there is some other emergency. Always use the correct equipment and, if necessary, get training from a qualified instructor to minimize your risk of injury. Never mix water sports and alcohol; more than 50 percent of boating accidents and drownings occur among people who have been drinking alcoholic beverages.

WARNING

If you participate in water activities, protect yourself against the weather. A strong, cold wind blowing on wet clothing can rapidly chill your body and may cause hypothermia, a potentially life-threatening condition in which the body temperature drops quickly. If you don't have dry clothes to change into, get out of the cold wind as quickly as possible. Also, avoid overexposure to heat, which can result in heat exhaustion (extreme weakness and partial dehydration) or heat stroke (extremely high fever and physical collapse). The risk of sunburn is much greater around water because the sun's ultraviolet rays are reflected up by the water's surface. Wear a shirt and apply a waterproof sunscreen to exposed areas of your skin.

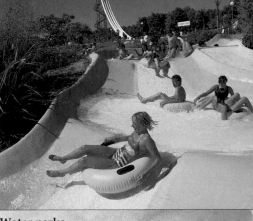

Water parks
A water park – an amusement park featuring water slides and wave pools – is good family fun. It's reasonably safe if you take a few precautions. Always be sure that there are trained lifeguards on duty. Children who have not yet learned how to swim should wear flotation devices. Read all signs that warn of dangers or risks of injury. Do not run near the water and follow the rules for going down the water slides.

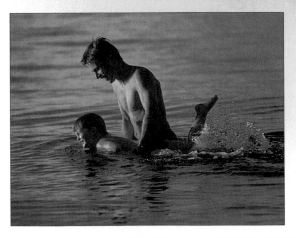

Scuba diving
Talk to your doctor before taking up scuba diving, particularly if you have a history of high blood pressure or heart disease. Make sure you are trained by a qualified instructor, that you know how to use the diving equipment properly, and that you follow safety procedures at all times (see page 110).

Swimming and diving
Never go swimming alone, and make sure children are supervised at all times. If you do not know how to swim, do not enter water that you cannot stand up in or shallow water that has a strong undertow. Make sure that you heed any warning flags or signs about safety rules and water conditions. Do not dive into the water unless you have checked the depth of the water.

Fishing

When you are fishing, keep a close eye on children; make sure they do not stand too close to the water, because riverbanks and lake shores may have unstable edges. Know the waters in which you fish. Weather changes can cause water conditions to become hazardous suddenly. Always check for flood warnings; a flood can cause a dangerously strong current in a slow-moving river or stream.

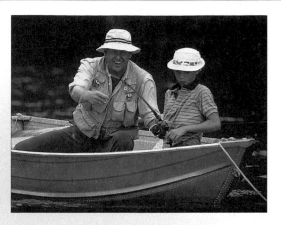

Sailboarding

Do not try sailboarding unless you have been trained and you are a good swimmer. Make sure you have sufficient strength and stamina to handle demanding wind and water conditions. Always wear a life jacket and protect your hands with gloves. Be aware of boats and watch out for swimmers close to the shore. Carry a small waterproof flare or smoke signal in case the wind takes you too far away from the shore.

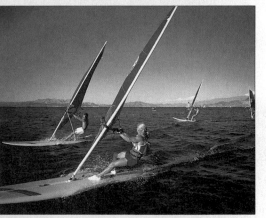

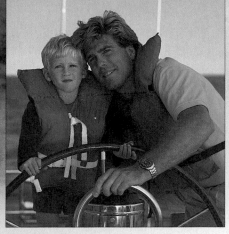

Boating

Check the weather conditions before you take a boat trip. Make sure you know the emergency procedures for an overboard passenger and for capsizing. Always wear a life jacket. For night sailing, the life jacket should have a whistle attached and a light that goes on automatically if you fall in the water.

EMERGENCY SUPPLIES FOR THE BOAT

In 1990, nearly 900 people died and almost 4,000 people were injured in boating accidents. If you are going boating, always be prepared for an emergency. Make sure that you have the following equipment aboard at all times:

◆ Life jackets (one per person)
◆ First-aid kit (see page 43)
◆ Life preserver with a throw rope
◆ Flares, a red smoke canister, and a mirror to signal for help
◆ Whistle
◆ Large container of fresh water
◆ Knife
◆ Waterproof matches
◆ Flashlight
◆ Two-way radio
◆ Emergency food supplies
◆ A water pump or bucket to bail water out of the boat
◆ Oars

Canoeing

Wear a snug-fitting, vest-type life jacket. Avoid bulky clothing that could reduce your ability to swim. If you are a beginner, take a class to learn the safety skills, such as how to handle your canoe and how to recognize common hazards. Make sure you are familiar with the body of water and check the weather conditions before taking a canoe trip.

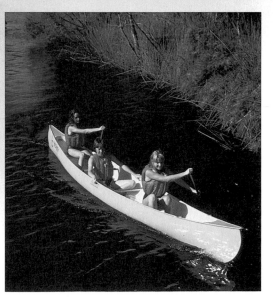

SPORTS CLOTHING AND SAFETY EQUIPMENT

You can avoid many sports or exercise injuries by wearing the appropriate clothing and using proper safety equipment. As experts learn more about the causes of injury, the makers of safety equipment have developed a wider variety of products that provide more effective protection. For example, the design of the back of football helmets has been altered to decrease the likelihood of injury to the neck. Many athletes now wear knee braces to decrease the possibility of damage to the knee joint. You can also protect yourself against injury by being aware of potential hazards. For example, runners should wear reflective clothing when running at night or in foggy weather and carry flashlights on dimly lit roads so that drivers can see them.

Clothing and shoes

Make sure your clothes are comfortable and that they provide adequate protection. Also, consider the weather if you work out outside. Wearing shoes that are designed specifically for your sport – and that fit properly – can help prevent foot and ankle injuries. For example, tennis shoes should not be used for running, nor should running shoes be used for playing tennis. A tennis shoe does not have the shock absorbency of a running shoe, and a running shoe does not provide enough support for the stop-and-go action needed in tennis. Running shoes lose their shock absorbency after about 500 miles of running, so make sure you replace your running shoes regularly or alternate between two or three pairs.

Safety equipment

Ask an expert to help you choose the most appropriate safety equipment for your activity and to demonstrate how to use the equipment correctly. Several types of safety goggles are available to protect your eyes from injury or irritation. Racquetball and handball players should always wear safety goggles to prevent eye injury. People who play racket sports should choose a racket with a handle size that is correct for their grip – the circumference of the handle should be equal to the distance between the tip of the middle finger and the middle of the palm. Mouth

Safety goggles
In some sports, safety goggles are recommended to prevent eye injury. Serious eye injuries and blindness have occurred as a result of a racquetball hitting the eye. Swimming and skiing goggles protect the eyes and prevent irritation.

guards are recommended for most contact sports. Shock-absorbing mats should be used with all gymnastic equipment.

Helmets are recommended for many sports, especially skateboarding, bicycling, and skating, in which the head is vulnerable to injury. Most helmets have a fiberglass or plastic outer shell and an inner lining of resilient material to absorb a single strong force (as in a fall when horseback riding or bicycling) or multiple forces caused by collisions (as in the physical contact that occurs during football). Select a helmet that has a sticker that certifies approval by a nationally known safety organization. Make sure that your helmet is the right size and, most important, that you wear it.

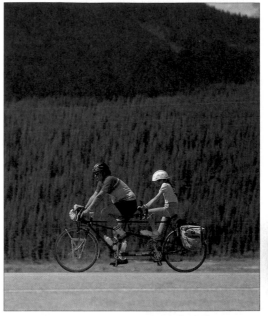

Helmets save lives
Always wear a helmet when riding a bicycle or motorcycle. About 75 percent of bicycle fatalities are caused by head injuries. A recent study showed that motorcyclists who were not wearing helmets had almost three times as many head injuries as those who wore helmets.

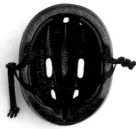

IS YOUR CHILD'S PLAYGROUND SAFE?

Most children spend their summer vacation playing outdoors, often at a nearby playground. About 185,000 children require treatment every year at hospital emergency departments for injuries that occur on playgrounds. Most of these injuries are caused by falls from climbing equipment such as monkey bars and chin-up bars. Other injuries at playgrounds occur when children are hit by moving equipment or when they fall against protruding hardware or onto a hard surface. The following tips can help protect your child from injury at his or her playground.

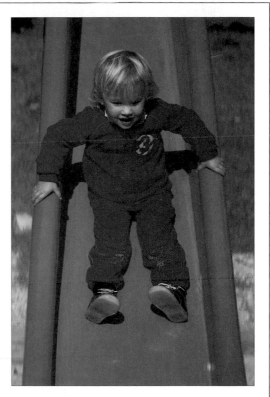

Play it safe
You can help reduce your child's risk of injury at the playground by showing him or her how to use the equipment safely. Teach your child not to walk too close in front or back of moving swings. Show your child how to climb up the rungs of the slide, one at a time and holding on to the handrails, and to slide down feet first. Tell your child not to play on playground equipment that is wet, icy, or very hot.

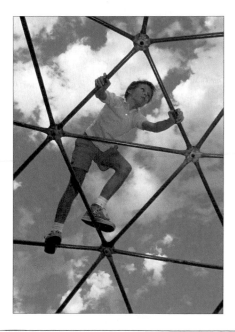

◆ Check the equipment at your child's playground for components that form angles or openings that could trap your child's head.

◆ Make sure that there are no sharp edges that could cut or puncture skin or entangle your child's clothing.

◆ Be sure the playground is surfaced with shock-absorbent materials (such as wood chips, sand, or pea-sized gravel) to help prevent injury from a fall.

DRIVING SAFELY

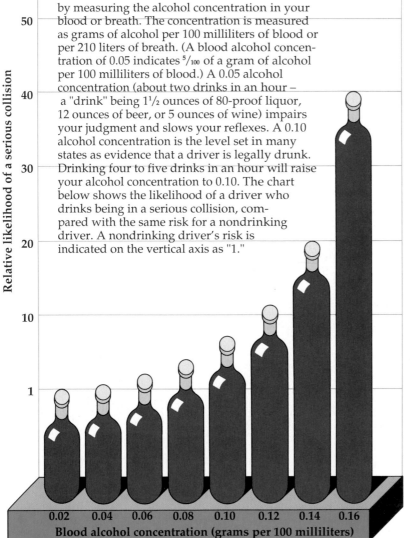

Drinking and driving
Law enforcement officers establish intoxication by measuring the alcohol concentration in your blood or breath. The concentration is measured as grams of alcohol per 100 milliliters of blood or per 210 liters of breath. (A blood alcohol concentration of 0.05 indicates $5/100$ of a gram of alcohol per 100 milliliters of blood.) A 0.05 alcohol concentration (about two drinks in an hour – a "drink" being 1½ ounces of 80-proof liquor, 12 ounces of beer, or 5 ounces of wine) impairs your judgment and slows your reflexes. A 0.10 alcohol concentration is the level set in many states as evidence that a driver is legally drunk. Drinking four to five drinks in an hour will raise your alcohol concentration to 0.10. The chart below shows the likelihood of a driver who drinks being in a serious collision, compared with the same risk for a nondrinking driver. A nondrinking driver's risk is indicated on the vertical axis as "1."

Relative likelihood of a serious collision (vertical axis: 1, 10, 20, 30, 40, 50, 60)

Blood alcohol concentration (grams per 100 milliliters) (horizontal axis: 0.02, 0.04, 0.06, 0.08, 0.10, 0.12, 0.14, 0.16)

Motor-vehicle accidents are the leading cause of accidental death. Nearly 47,000 people die in motor-vehicle accidents every year. For every death, four people are seriously injured, many of whom are left with permanent disabilities.

Collision between vehicles is the most common type of accident in both rural and urban areas. In fatal two-vehicle collisions, collision at an angle is most prevalent in urban areas and head-on collision is most common in rural areas. Use of seat belts is critical in a collision. In a head-on collision at 30 miles per hour, your car would begin to slow down and the front end would crush on impact, absorbing some of the force of the collision. The car would come to a complete stop within one tenth of a second. About one fiftieth of a second later, a driver who was not wearing a seat belt would still be moving inside the car at 30 miles per hour and would hit the windshield or steering wheel like a missile.

FACTORS IN ROAD SAFETY

Driver error is the major cause of collisions. Safe driving is important in preventing motor-vehicle accidents, no matter how far you are driving – whether you are just going to the store or driving a long distance. Most motor-vehicle accidents occur within 5 miles of home.

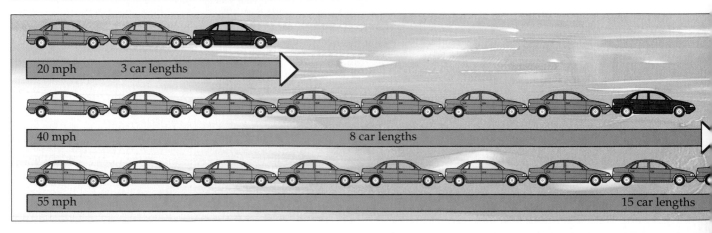

20 mph — 3 car lengths

40 mph — 8 car lengths

55 mph — 15 car lengths

Seat belts

Using a lap and shoulder belt in your vehicle reduces the risk of serious or fatal injuries by between 40 and 55 percent. The number of drivers who use seat belts has increased from about 11 percent in 1982 to 49 percent in 1990. From 1983 to 1989, use of seat belts saved an estimated 20,000 lives and prevented about 520,000 moderate to severe injuries. Statistics for the period 1982 through 1989 show that seat belt use among drinking drivers who were involved in fatal crashes was less than that among nondrinking drivers. In cars that have automatic shoulder restraint systems, an occupant is still at high risk of serious or fatal injury if the lap belt is not used in conjunction with the shoulder apparatus.

Alcohol and other drugs

Never drink and drive. Alcohol impairs your judgment and coordination and slows your reflexes. People are affected differently from drinking the same amount of alcohol. The effects of alcohol are influenced by factors such as your body weight, the amount of alcohol you drank, the time elapsed since your last drink, your mental and physical condition, the amount and type of food you've eaten, and the presence of other drugs in your body. Nearly 50 percent of drivers who are killed every year drink alcohol before their accident. Of these, 80 percent had a blood alcohol concentration above 0.10 – the level at which many states consider a driver to be intoxicated. Some medications (such as antihistamines and tranquilizers) and all drugs of abuse impair your ability to drive safely.

Speed

A vehicle traveling at 60 miles per hour has nine times the kinetic energy (the energy derived from its movement) as the same vehicle traveling at 20 miles per hour. The probability of being seriously injured in a motor-vehicle accident is three times higher when driving at 55 miles per hour than at 25 miles per hour; the probability of being killed in a motor-vehicle accident is five times higher at 55 miles per hour than at 25 miles per hour.

Defensive driving

Always drive defensively. Maintain a safe distance between your car and the car ahead of you and drive at a speed that is appropriate to the road and weather conditions. The faster your car is traveling and the heavier the car, the longer it takes to stop. Wet driving conditions increase the distance you need to stop your car safely. Some estimated average stopping distances are shown below. Never assume another driver will yield the right of way, watch for and avoid hazards such as drunk drivers, and avoid a driver's blind spot behind his or her car. To brush up on or improve your driving skills, you can enroll in a defensive driving course. These courses are offered by the National Safety Council.

Car safety: check it yourself
Make safety checks on your vehicle in the spring and fall.

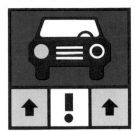

Check for burned-out lights at the front and rear of your vehicle.

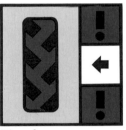

Tires that are worn should be replaced. If tires are losing their tread on one side, check your wheel alignment.

Replace worn-out windshield wiper blades, and periodically check and refill the windshield washer fluid.

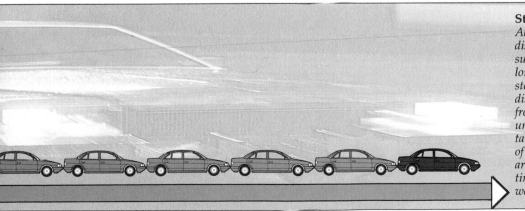

Stopping distance
Always maintain a safe stopping distance. Stopping distance is the sum of your reaction distance (how long it takes to see a hazard and step on the brake) plus the braking distance (how far your car travels from the time you step on the brake until the car stops). Braking distance is influenced by the weight of your car, the speed at which you are traveling, the condition of your tires and brakes, and the road and weather conditions.

A SAFER AUTOMOBILE

Today's automobiles offer a variety of safety features. While some features are standard, others are available as options. Car manufacturers develop safety systems to protect the occupants of the car in the event of a collision and to reduce the effects of a collision on the car itself. Make sure your car is in good working condition and that all safety features work properly. When buying a new car, ask about the safety features that are available, and be sure to select a car that has a good rating for safety on the road.

SAFETY FEATURES

A large, heavy car provides good protection. In the event of a collision, there is more room around you in the passenger compartment. Many people today drive small, compact cars because they are economical, maneuverable, and easy to park. However, these cars offer less protection in an accident because you are seated closer to the car's interior surfaces.

Steering wheels
Many drivers are injured when they are propelled forward into the steering wheel in a collision. An anti-intrusion system can be fitted to the steering column to reduce the distance that the steering column and wheel can be forced into the passenger compartment in a head-on collision. Padded and collapsible steering wheels are also available.

Crush zones
Many vehicles absorb some of the impact of a collision by crushing in predetermined areas – called crush zones – at the front and rear of a vehicle. Crush zones are designed so that the passenger compartment of a vehicle is the last area to be affected by a collision.

Head rests
Head rests reduce the risk of neck injury occurring as a result of a rear impact. The head rest should be positioned behind the middle of your head. A head rest that is too low can make a neck injury worse.

Seat belts
A seat belt should lie high on your shoulder and across your pelvis, rather than your stomach. Infants and small children must sit in safety seats (see CAR TRIPS *on page 20).*

Childproof locks
Childproof locks on car windows and rear doors are designed to prevent injury (see page 20).

Air bags

Air bags provide extra protection when used along with seat belts. An air bag inflates upon impact in a head-on collision and prevents you from hitting your head on the steering wheel or windshield (see sequence at far right).

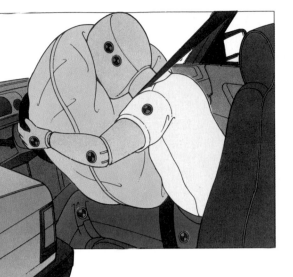

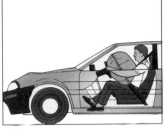

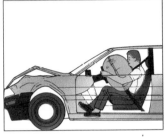

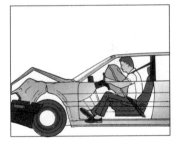

Rear brake light
A high, centrally mounted, rear brake light provides an easily visible signal to drivers behind you.

Antilock brakes
The efficiency of brakes drops considerably once the wheels are locked and skidding on the road surface. Antilock-braking systems are designed to stop a car without locking the wheels, preventing your car from skidding and allowing you to steer the car to avoid a collision.

CAR TROUBLE? WHAT TO DO IN AN EMERGENCY

Driving emergencies can result from sudden mechanical failure, even in a well-maintained vehicle. If you have a flat tire or need to make an emergency stop for any reason, drive off the roadway and onto the shoulder; never stop in traffic lanes. Always get out of your car on the passenger side – away from the flow of traffic.

Sticking gas pedal
Tap your foot on the gas pedal two or three times or try to pull the pedal up with the toe of your shoe. If the pedal remains stuck, shift the transmission into neutral and apply the brakes.

Brake failure
Rapidly pump the brakes to restore pressure in the brake line. If this does not work, put the car in a lower gear and slowly apply the parking brake.

Engine fire
Pull off the road, turn off the engine, and get everyone out of the car immediately. If possible, use a rag to open the hood and try to put out the fire with a fire extinguisher or blanket.

Stalling engine
Do not turn off the ignition – this may cause the steering to lock. Shift the transmission into neutral and steer your car off the roadway and onto the shoulder.

Overheating engine
Pull off the road and turn off the engine; let it cool for at least 15 minutes. Use a rag to remove the radiator cap (beware of escaping steam); add warm water while the engine is running.

Loss of steering
While you brake to bring your car to a stop, sound your horn and turn on your emergency flashers to warn pedestrians and other drivers.

CHAPTER TWO

EMERGENCY PROCEDURES

EMERGENCY FIRST AID is immediate treatment given to a person with an injury or sudden illness. If properly administered within the first few minutes after an accident, emergency first aid can make the difference between life and death. The main objectives of emergency first aid are to prevent the person's condition from worsening, to protect the person from further injury, to provide immediate care that allows the person to recover from the injury, to provide reassurance to the person, and to make the person as comfortable as possible until medical personnel arrive.

If you were to witness a medical emergency, would you know what to do? Knowing what to do and reacting quickly and calmly enable you to provide the best care to an accident victim. Your actions may also help medical personnel to provide care more effectively once they arrive.

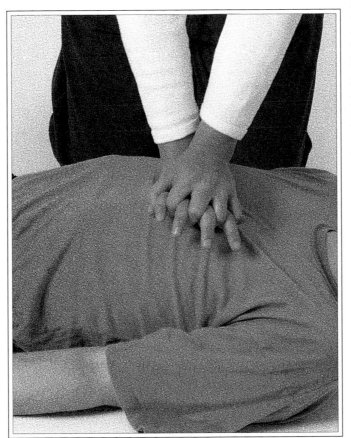

Many injuries require the common-sense first-aid measures we learned as children. However, some injuries and medical emergencies are life-threatening and require more advanced first-aid skills. This chapter gives guidelines and instructions on immediate first-aid treatment for several life-threatening emergencies, such as a heart attack, choking, shock, and severe bleeding.

The first section provides information on training in emergency first aid, discusses the emergency telephone numbers and medical information you should have handy in case of an emergency, and tells you what you should do if you are the first person to arrive at the scene of an accident. The section on emergency resuscitation explains how to determine whether someone has stopped breathing or had a cardiac arrest (cessation of heartbeat). Instructions are given on how to revive a person who has stopped breathing and how to perform cardiopulmonary resuscitation to restore circulation if the heart has stopped beating. For each emergency first-aid procedure, the different techniques that are used to resuscitate infants, children, and adults are described. We also describe the proper technique for relieving obstruction of the airway in a person who is choking. The section on immediate first aid for bleeding and shock provides information on how to evaluate the severity of bleeding and how to recognize the symptoms of shock. Also included are instructions on how to administer emergency first aid to an injury victim who is bleeding severely. The final section explains the procedures for emergency childbirth. As you prepare for a baby's arrival, remember that most births occur naturally and normally.

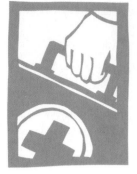

BE PREPARED

KNOWING HOW TO PROVIDE the proper first-aid care for emergencies saves lives. If you are trained in first-aid you will be able to recognize the signs and symptoms of a heart attack, perform artificial ventilation and cardiopulmonary resuscitation, help someone who is choking, and prevent an accident victim from being injured further until medical help arrives. Don't wait until accidents happen to learn these skills; be prepared.

Emergency training
Qualified first-aid training centers are equipped with mannequins on which you can practice techniques such as artificial ventilation and cardiopulmonary resuscitation. The chest of the mannequin (below right) rises when the artificial ventilation technique is performed correctly.

Taking safety precautions reduces the risk of accidental injury, but not all accidents can be prevented. Fortunately, most accidents result in minor injuries such as small cuts or bruises. It is important that you be fully prepared and know how to react if you or the people around you become involved in a serious emergency. The action taken within the first few minutes after an accident often determines whether a person will survive a potentially fatal injury.

EMERGENCY FIRST AID

Being trained in first aid helps to ensure that your actions will have the desired results. Learn to recognize possible signs of a heart attack (see page 49) and know how to administer cardiopulmonary resuscitation (CPR). If you begin CPR promptly on a person having a heart attack, you can save his or her life. In a major study in Seattle, 175,000 residents received basic training in CPR. In 1 year, 43 percent of victims survived after CPR was administered by a bystander, compared to 21 percent when emergency first-aid was delayed until medical help arrived. Groups such as the American Red Cross offer first-aid courses and information. Once you learn first-aid techniques, you should take a refresher course every 2 years.

FIRST-AID KIT

A first-aid kit should contain the basic items required in an emergency. Keep a first-aid kit at home and in your car and take a first-aid kit with you on vacations. Check the contents regularly and remember to replace used items. Before going on vacation, call your doctor for prescription medications that you or members of your family may require.

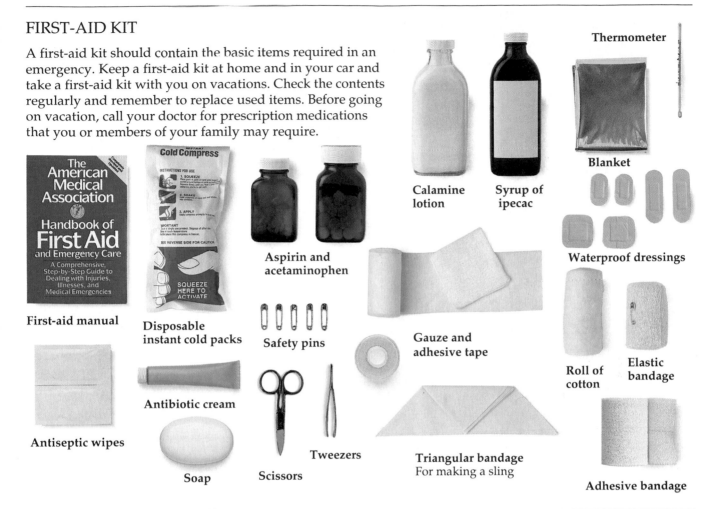

First-aid manual

Disposable instant cold packs

Safety pins

Aspirin and acetaminophen

Calamine lotion

Syrup of ipecac

Thermometer

Blanket

Waterproof dressings

Gauze and adhesive tape

Antiseptic wipes

Antibiotic cream

Soap

Scissors

Tweezers

Triangular bandage
For making a sling

Roll of cotton

Elastic bandage

Adhesive bandage

Knowing where to call

Post the telephone number and location of your local poison control center and hospital emergency department near the telephone. Use the 911 phone number or other type of emergency response system available in your community to call for an ambulance. If you call for an ambulance, give your name, location, and telephone number; then briefly explain what has happened and describe any obvious injuries. Remain calm and follow all the instructions you are given. If possible, have someone watch for the ambulance and direct the medical personnel to the victim. Depending on the type and severity of the injury or illness and the level of emergency medical services available in your community, taking your own car to the hospital may be quicker than waiting for an ambulance. If possible, call ahead to the emergency department to tell the medical personnel that you are on the way and the type of illness or injury that has occurred.

Emergency information

Keep a record of the medical history of each member of your family. Make a note of when immunizations are given, of medications being taken (including dosages), and of any allergies (such as to insect bites or medications).

Medical information is particularly important if you have a medical condition such as diabetes or hemophilia. Wearing a bracelet or necklace with emergency information on it, or carrying this information on a card in your wallet, could save your life if you are injured and are unable to speak. Your identification information should contain your name and address and any medical condition or allergy you have.

WARNING

Call an ambulance if a person shows any of the following signs or symptoms:

◆ Severe bleeding
◆ Loss or decreased level of consciousness
◆ Severe abdominal pain
◆ Difficulty breathing
◆ Severe chest pain
◆ Shortness of breath
◆ Seizure lasting 5 or more minutes
◆ Signs of cardio-vascular collapse (cold or clammy skin or impaired responsiveness)

WHAT SHOULD I DO AT THE SCENE OF AN ACCIDENT?

If you are the first person at the scene of an accident, quickly evaluate the situation before taking action. While it is important to help an injured person, do not attempt to do so if it means placing yourself in danger. If you are alone at the scene, administer the necessary first aid for any immediately life-threatening injury before calling for medical help.

1 If the person's injuries have resulted from a fall or motor-vehicle accident, do not move the person unless it is absolutely necessary. Moving an injured person could make a back or neck injury worse and could cause paralysis.

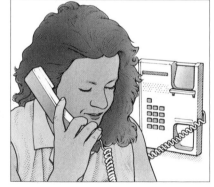

4 Call for help or ask someone else to call for medical assistance. Calling 911 (or the emergency number for your community) early is vital so that medical personnel can get to the scene as quickly as possible; ask if there is any more you can do until they arrive.

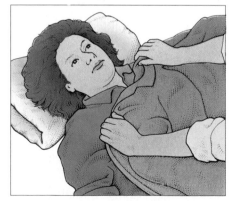

5 Loosen tight clothing and cover the person with a coat or blanket. In most cases, the person should lie down or, at least, recline.

6 Gather facts from other people at the scene. Give all information to medical personnel when they arrive. Obtaining information about the events leading up to an accident can be crucial. For example, knowing that a driver had severe chest pains and passed out before an accident suggests that the person has a medical condition in addition to any injuries caused by the accident.

2 If the person is in an unsafe environment (such as near a fire), try to move the person to a safe place, taking extra care to move the spine as little as possible.

3 Assess the injuries and attend to the most seriously injured persons first. If the person is unconscious, perform the ABCs of basic life support (see right).

HAZARDS TO YOUR SAFETY

Do not approach an accident victim if doing so endangers your life; prevent others from doing so. If possible, eliminate the danger. If an accident victim must be moved, immobilize all parts of the body before doing so.

Never touch a person who is in contact with electricity. Try to turn off the electricity or use a dry board or wood-handled broom to move the person out of contact with the electricity.

Do not approach a vehicle carrying toxic chemicals that has been involved in an accident. Protective clothing may be required for rescue efforts.

Fire or a danger of explosion may indicate that you should not approach the accident scene until the danger has been eliminated. However, if a person has had a heart attack and has suffered cardiac arrest, try to quickly move the person to safety and administer CPR (see page 50).

Watch for moving objects such as traffic or falling debris at the scene of an accident.

To help a drowning person, reach out from the bank, shore, or edge of pool, throw a life preserver, or row out to the person (see page 108).

ABCs OF BASIC LIFE SUPPORT

The letters "ABC" are a simple way to remember the three steps you should take in an emergency if you think a person is not breathing. These letters stand for airway, breathing, and circulation.

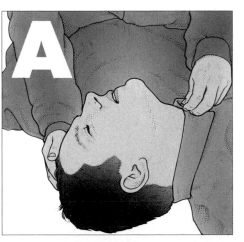

Airway
To open the airway, use the head tilt/ chin lift technique. (If a neck injury is suspected, do not twist or rotate the person's head.) Place the palm of one hand on the person's forehead and the fingers of your other hand under the bony part of the person's chin; tilt the head back.

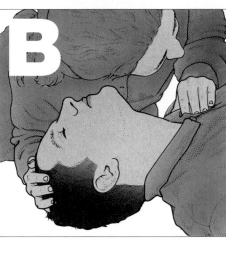

Breathing
Check to see if the person is breathing. Kneel down beside the injured person to look for movements of the chest, to hear air being exhaled, and to feel for breath. If the person is not breathing, perform artificial ventilation (see page 47).

Circulation
If the person is breathing, the heart is beating. If the person is not breathing and does not quickly respond to artificial ventilation, check for a pulse (see page 49). If there is no pulse, tell someone to call for medical assistance and begin CPR (see page 50).

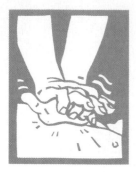

EMERGENCY RESUSCITATION

ARTIFICIAL VENTILATION and cardiopulmonary resuscitation (CPR) are basic lifesaving techniques that can be used to help a person whose breathing or heartbeat has stopped. These techniques allow you to mimic the actions normally performed by the heart and lungs in an attempt to circulate blood and oxygen.

If a person has collapsed and is unconscious, follow the ABCs of basic life support (outlined on page 45). Check the airway (A), restore breathing (B), and restore circulation (C) – these are the three basic steps involved in resuscitation. For a person who is not breathing but has a heartbeat, check the airway for obstruction and perform artificial ventilation if necessary (see page 47). A person who is not breathing and whose heart has also stopped beating requires cardiopulmonary resuscitation (CPR), which consists of artificial ventilation and chest compressions (see page 50).

OPENING THE AIRWAY

Some common causes of breathing emergencies include airway obstruction, ingestion of poisonous substances, injury to the chest or lungs, heart attack, near-drowning, electrocution, and reactions to insect bites or stings.

If a person is not breathing, there will be no up-and-down movement of the chest or abdomen and you will not be able to hear or feel air being exhaled. To make sure, kneel down next to the person and turn your head so that your ear is just above his or her mouth and nose. If you cannot hear any breathing or feel any breath on your ear, attempt to restore breathing by opening the person's airway (use the head tilt/chin lift technique shown at left). If the airway is blocked by a foreign object, clear the airway as described on page 52; do not attempt this procedure on a child unless you can see the obstructing object.

If the person having breathing difficulties has a head or neck injury, the part of the spine in the neck area may also be injured; the neck and head should be moved as little as possible. However, the airway takes priority; you must open the airway and supply artificial ventilation if necessary. For techniques to immobilize the neck area, see page 73.

UPPER AIRWAY OBSTRUCTION

Breathing problems in an unconscious person are often caused by obstruction of the airway by the tongue. Pushing the person's head back elevates the tongue away from the base of the throat. Artificial ventilation (see page 47) may be required if the person is not breathing.

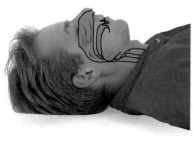

Breathing problems
The tongue has fallen to the back of the throat, blocking the airway.

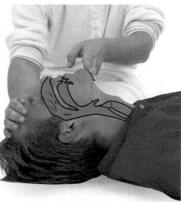

Head tilt/chin lift
Tilt the head back by gently pushing the forehead back and lifting the chin; this reopens the airway and allows breathing to resume.

ARTIFICIAL VENTILATION

Artificial ventilation is an emergency procedure used to restore breathing. The method of artificial ventilation used most often is mouth-to-mouth resuscitation. If a person is not breathing and no neck injury is suspected, perform all of the following four steps. If a neck injury is suspected, do not twist or rotate the head. Elevate the chin slightly to open the airway.

MOUTH-TO-MOUTH RESUSCITATION

1 Make sure the person is on a firm, rigid surface such as the floor. Place the palm of one hand on the person's forehead and the fingers of your other hand under the bony part of the person's chin and tilt the head back.

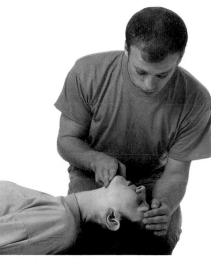

2 Pinch the person's nostrils closed using your thumb and index finger. Open your mouth wide and take a deep breath. Be sure not to obstruct the person's throat with your supporting hand.

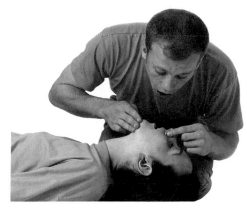

3 Place your open mouth tightly over the person's mouth and give two full breaths of 1 to 1¹/₂ seconds each. Remove your mouth after each exhalation and take a deep breath between each one.

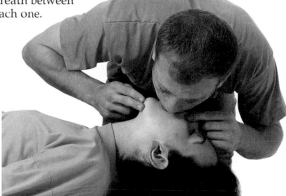

4 Turn your head toward the person's chest so that your ear is over his or her mouth. Listen for air being exhaled. Watch for the person's chest to fall. Continue blowing into the person's mouth at a rate of 12 breaths per minute for an adult or 15 breaths per minute for a child. Continue until the person begins to breathe on his or her own or medical help arrives.

RESUSCITATING AN INFANT

1 If an infant is not breathing, tilt the infant's head back. To open the airway, press gently on the forehead with the palm of one hand. Place the finger tips of the other hand on the bony part of the jaw near the chin and lift upward. Do not extend the infant's head back too far because you may close the airway.

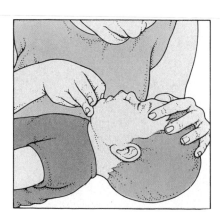

2 Place your mouth tightly over the infant's mouth and nose and blow two breaths so that the infant's chest rises. Do not blow air as forcefully as for an adult. Blow gently into the lungs at a rate of one breath every 3 seconds.

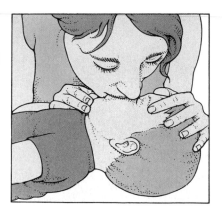

MOUTH-TO-NOSE RESUSCITATION

In some cases, mouth-to-mouth resuscitation is not possible. For example, the person may have a mouth injury or a jaw that cannot be opened. In such instances, use mouth-to-nose resuscitation to restore breathing.

1 Place the palm of one hand on the person's forehead and tilt the person's head back. With the fingers of your other hand, close the person's mouth and lift the chin. If a neck injury is suspected, do not twist or rotate the head; elevate the chin slightly to open the airway.

2 Take a deep breath, then seal your mouth around the person's nose. Breathe two full breaths into the nose.

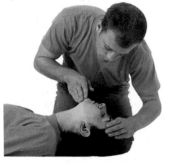

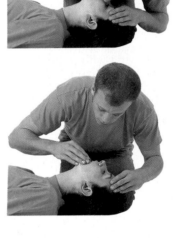

3 Open the person's mouth to allow air to escape. Continue at a rate of 12 breaths per minute until the person begins to breathe on his or her own or medical help arrives.

BREATHING AND CIRCULATION

To maintain life, the human body needs to take in oxygen and eliminate carbon dioxide – a process called respiration. Both breathing and the pumping of blood around the body by the heart are vital to the exchange of oxygen and carbon dioxide by your cells (see below). Oxygen in the air breathed into the lungs enters the blood; this oxygen-rich blood is carried from the lungs to the heart, which then pumps blood through the arteries to all parts of the body. The oxygen then moves from the blood into the cells and carbon dioxide is taken up in exchange. The blood, now depleted of oxygen but rich in carbon dioxide, is returned to the heart by the veins. The heart pumps the blood to the lungs, where carbon dioxide is exhaled and oxygen is inhaled to complete the cycle of respiration. If breathing stops and the heart stops beating, oxygen cannot enter the blood and blood cannot be circulated. Death quickly results unless both breathing and circulation can be restored promptly.

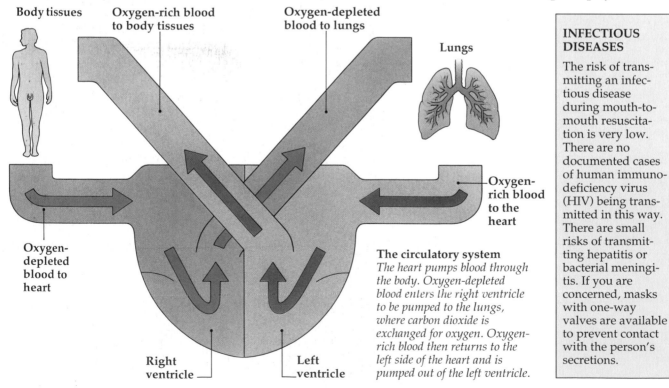

Body tissues

Oxygen-rich blood to body tissues

Oxygen-depleted blood to lungs

Lungs

Oxygen-rich blood to the heart

Oxygen-depleted blood to heart

Right ventricle

Left ventricle

The circulatory system
The heart pumps blood through the body. Oxygen-depleted blood enters the right ventricle to be pumped to the lungs, where carbon dioxide is exchanged for oxygen. Oxygen-rich blood then returns to the left side of the heart and is pumped out of the left ventricle.

INFECTIOUS DISEASES

The risk of transmitting an infectious disease during mouth-to-mouth resuscitation is very low. There are no documented cases of human immunodeficiency virus (HIV) being transmitted in this way. There are small risks of transmitting hepatitis or bacterial meningitis. If you are concerned, masks with one-way valves are available to prevent contact with the person's secretions.

CARDIAC ARREST

Cardiac arrest may be caused by a heart attack, cessation of breathing from any cause, an electric shock, severe loss of blood, poisoning, a drug overdose, severe hypothermia (see page 105), or anaphylactic shock (see page 117). Cardiac arrest occurs when the pumping action of the heart stops or is replaced with ineffective contraction of the large lower chambers of the heart. The latter is called ventricular fibrillation. Interference in the pumping action of the heart prevents blood from moving to all other areas of the body; the person stops breathing and collapses. The tissues of the body do not die immediately but begin to deteriorate as the oxygen supply decreases.

If you witness a cardiac arrest, the first 4 to 6 minutes are critical for efforts to revive the person and prevent perma-

WARNING SIGNS OF A HEART ATTACK

A heart attack occurs when one or more blood vessels that supply blood to the heart are blocked. This blockage of blood to the heart damages part of the heart muscle due to lack of oxygen. The warning signs of a heart attack are given below:

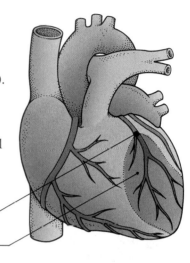

◆ Chest pain (pressure, squeezing, fullness or tightness in the center of the chest or upper part of the abdomen).
◆ Pain that may spread to the shoulders or arms or to the neck, jaw, and back.
◆ Sweating, nausea, abnormal paleness, shortness of breath, dizziness, or fainting.

Blocked coronary artery

Damaged heart muscle

Checking an adult's pulse
To check for a pulse, move two fingers along the person's throat to the Adam's apple. Then move these fingers to the side of the person's throat between the windpipe and the muscles at the side of the neck and press down firmly.

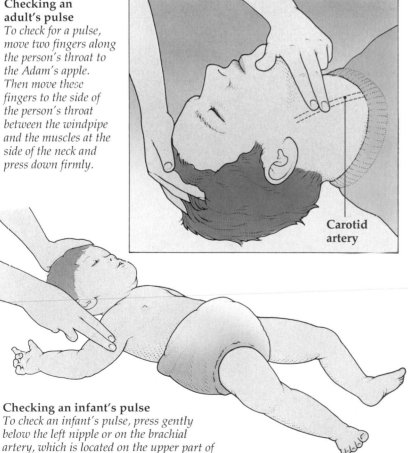

Carotid artery

Checking an infant's pulse
To check an infant's pulse, press gently below the left nipple or on the brachial artery, which is located on the upper part of the arm between the elbow and the shoulder.

nent damage. After that time, irreversible damage to the brain may occur so that the person cannot be revived (this state is known as brain death). Administer CPR (see page 50) until medical personnel trained in advanced life-support techniques, such as defibrillation, intravenous medication, or airway intubation techniques, arrive.

CHECKING THE HEARTBEAT

Before starting CPR, you must make sure that the victim has had a cardiac arrest and that he or she has not simply fainted. If a person's heart has stopped beating, you will be unable to feel a pulse at the wrist or neck, and you will not hear a heartbeat in the person's chest. If a person is breathing, then the heart is beating, even if you cannot feel a pulse. You can check for a pulse in one of the carotid arteries on either side of the victim's neck (see left). If you feel a pulse, the heart is beating; if you do not feel a pulse, begin CPR immediately.

CARDIOPULMONARY RESUSCITATION

Cardiopulmonary resuscitation (CPR) is a lifesaving technique performed to restore breathing and circulation in a person whose heart has stopped beating and who is not breathing. It is vital to restore circulation of oxygen-carrying blood to the brain as quickly as possible because permanent brain damage or death is likely if oxygen is cut off for more than 4 to 6 minutes. CPR works by simulating the pumping action of the heart, while at the same time providing oxygen to the lungs.

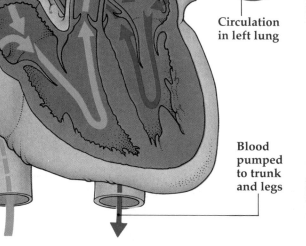

Blood pumped to head and arms

Circulation in right lung

Circulation in left lung

Blood pumped to trunk and legs

WARNING

CPR should be performed only after thorough training in the procedure. Inexpert application of the technique may be harmful to the person – possibly causing fractured ribs or even rupture of the heart; wait for trained personnel to arrive. If your community does not offer a course in CPR, call your local heart association or the American Red Cross. Remember that CPR is a temporary life-sustaining technique and is not likely to restore effective functioning of the heart. If a cardiac arrest victim is to be saved, it is crucial to call for medical assistance so that advanced life-support care is initiated as soon as possible. However, once you have started CPR, do not stop (even if the person is not responding) until medical personnel take over.

How CPR works
If CPR is successful, the external chest compressions exert sufficient pressure on the lower half of the breastbone to increase the pressure inside the chest, forcing blood out of the heart and into the arteries. Releasing the pressure after each compression allows the heart to refill with blood. This artificial pumping action allows blood to circulate from the heart to other parts of the body.

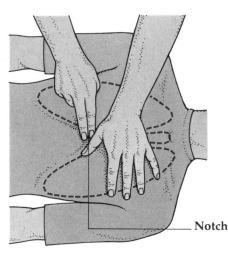

Notch

1 Kneel near the person's chest. With two fingers, locate the person's rib cage on the side closest to you. Move your fingers up the center of the chest to the notch where the ribs meet the breastbone. Keep two fingers on this notch and place the heel of your other hand two finger-widths above your fingers. Remove your fingers from the notch and place this hand on top of your other hand. Your fingers should be interlaced. (See also FINGER POSITIONS FOR INFANTS AND CHILDREN on the next page.)

2 Straighten your arms and lock your elbows. Use the heel of only one hand for the compressions. Push down (quickly and forcefully to a depth of 1¹/₂ to 2 inches) on the chest 15 times. Let the chest rise after each compression, but do not remove your hands from the chest. (For an infant or a child under 8, perform five compressions to a depth of 1 to 1¹/₂ inches.) Perform the technique rhythmically by counting "one and two and, three and four and, five and six and," and so on. Do not rock back and forth or sit on your heels because blood will not be pumped effectively.

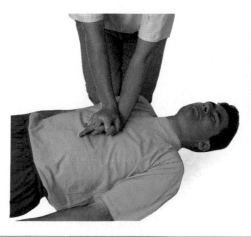

3 Remove your hands from the person's chest and open the airway by tilting the chin and head backward. Pinch the person's nostrils shut with your thumb and index finger. Blow two full breaths into his or her mouth so that the chest rises. (For a child under 8, blow one full breath only. For an infant, blow one full breath into the mouth and nose.)

VOMITING

If vomiting occurs during CPR, turn the person on his or her side (rolling the body as a single unit) and clear the mouth with your fingers. Return the person to his or her back and tilt the head back to open the airway. Resume mouth-to-mouth resuscitation and CPR, if necessary.

With two rescuers
If two rescuers are available, one rescuer performs chest compressions at a rate of 80 to 100 per minute, pausing after every fifth compression so that the second rescuer can give one slow breath. The second rescuer checks frequently for a pulse to ensure that the compressions are adequate to pump blood.

4 Reposition your hands on the chest and repeat the 15 compressions and two breaths. Perform four cycles of 15 compressions and two breaths and then determine if the pulse has returned (four cycles should take approximately 1 minute). For a child or an infant, perform 10 cycles of five compressions and one breath and then feel for a pulse. Do not stop CPR for longer than 7 seconds.

FINGER POSITIONS FOR INFANTS AND CHILDREN

For an infant, tilt the head back with the palm of your hand. With your other hand, draw an imaginary line between the nipples on the breastbone. Place two fingers one finger-width below this line on the breastbone; use these fingers to perform the compressions.

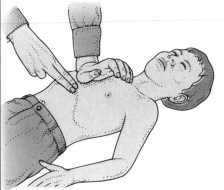

For children under age 8, move your fingers up the center of the child's chest to the notch where the ribs meet the breastbone. With your fingers on this notch, place the heel of your other hand two finger-widths above your fingers. Remove your fingers from the notch. Use one hand for chest compressions.

5 (Not shown.) Continue CPR until a pulse returns or medical help arrives. If a pulse returns, but breathing does not resume, perform artificial ventilation at 12 breaths per minute for an adult, 15 breaths per minute for a child, and 20 breaths per minute for an infant.

THE HEIMLICH MANEUVER

THE HEIMLICH MANEUVER is an emergency procedure that is designed to expel an obstruction from the airway of a person who is choking. In 1989, it is estimated that 3,900 people suffocated after food or other objects blocked the passage of air into their lungs. Prompt use of the Heimlich maneuver to remove the blockage could have prevented some of these deaths.

The airway, the passage by which air enters the lungs, must be open to allow breathing to occur. Choking results from an obstruction of the airway, either in the throat, the windpipe (trachea), or the air passages into the lungs (bronchi).

CHOKING

Food, liquids, or an inhaled or swallowed foreign object can cause choking. In children, choking is usually caused by a small piece of food such as a piece of popcorn or a peanut "going down the wrong way" and entering the trachea. If a person who is choking can speak, cough, or breathe, the blockage of the airway is only partial and you should not interfere. Allow the person to cough out the object on his or her own.

If the person cannot breathe and is unable to speak, there is likely to be a total blockage of the airway that must be quickly removed to prevent suffocation. The Heimlich maneuver (see page 53) produces an artificial cough to help a child or adult who is choking force the obstructing object out of the trachea.

If coughing is prolonged or the Heimlich maneuver does not successfully open the obstructed airway, call an ambulance or take the person to the nearest hospital emergency department.

WARNING

Victims of respiratory emergencies should be taken promptly to the nearest hospital emergency department. These emergencies include those caused by epiglottitis (inflammation of the flap of tissue at the back of the throat that closes off the windpipe during swallowing), a severe episode of asthma, pneumonia, inhalation of carbon monoxide or fumes from harmful chemicals, and acute bronchitis.

Clearing the airway
Grasp the person's lower jaw and tongue between the thumb and fingers of one hand and lift up the jaw. Check for any foreign material (such as food) that may be obstructing the airway. With the person's face up, insert your index finger down inside the cheek toward the base of the tongue. Move your finger across the back of the throat, using a "sweeping" motion to dislodge and remove any foreign material. Make sure you do not push an object farther down the throat. Check breathing again. Do not sweep the mouth of a child unless the foreign material is visible.

HOW TO PERFORM THE HEIMLICH MANEUVER

CONSCIOUS CHOKING VICTIM

1 Stand behind the person. Put your arms around the person's waist. Place your fist with the thumb side against the person's stomach above the navel and below the ribs and breastbone.

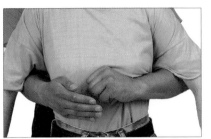

2 Hold your fist with your other hand and give four quick, forceful, upward and inward thrusts. Do not squeeze the ribs with your arms – use only your fist.

3 It may be necessary to repeat this movement six to 10 times. Continue until the person coughs up the object or becomes unconscious.

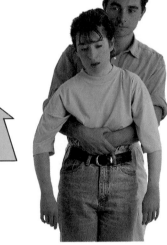

UNCONSCIOUS CHOKING VICTIM

1 Place the heel of one hand on the stomach, slightly above the navel and below the ribs. Put your free hand on top of your other hand. Keep your elbows straight. Give four quick, forceful, downward and forward thrusts toward the head.

2 If this method fails, try to remove the obstruction with your index finger (see CLEARING THE AIRWAY on page 52).

3 Repeat all of these steps as necessary until the object has been dislodged or medical help arrives.

Chest thrusts
If a choking victim is very overweight or pregnant, you may not be able to perform the Heimlich maneuver. If using the Heimlich maneuver is not possible, perform chest thrusts to remove an airway obstruction. Stand behind the person and place your arms under the person's armpits and around the chest. Place the thumb side of your fist on the middle of the breastbone. Grasp your fist with your other hand. Give four quick, forceful upward and inward thrusts. Do not squeeze your arms; use only your fists.

HOW TO REVIVE A CHOKING INFANT

1 Place the infant face down across your forearm with his or her head lower than the chest. Support the head by firmly holding the jaw. Rest your forearm on your thigh and give four forceful back blows between the shoulder blades with the heel of your hand.

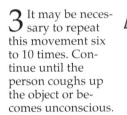

2 If unsuccessful, turn the baby over and, using two fingers, give four quick thrusts to the chest.

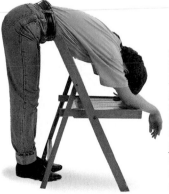

Self-administered Heimlich maneuver
If you are alone and are choking, place your fist on your stomach slightly above your navel and below your ribs. Put your other hand on top of your fist. Give four quick, forceful upward and inward thrusts. If this procedure does not work, press your stomach forcefully over a chair.

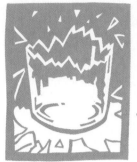

TREATMENT OF BLEEDING AND SHOCK

WHEN A PERSON is seriously injured, severe bleeding is a common cause of shock – a condition in which the blood pressure falls, the pulse becomes faster and weaker, and an inadequate amount of blood reaches the organs and tissues. Giving the appropriate first aid promptly can help control bleeding and prevent or reduce the severity of shock.

WARNING

Tourniquets can damage nerves and blood vessels and may stop the blood flow and cause the loss of a limb. They should be used only in extreme situations (see CONTROLLING BLEEDING on page 55).

Your heart pumps blood throughout your body in vessels called arteries. Capillaries, the smallest vessels, deliver blood to your organs and tissues. Your veins return blood to the heart. Bleeding occurs when these blood vessels are cut or torn. External bleeding occurs with open wounds such as cuts, lacerations, abrasions, and punctures. Bleeding can also occur internally. For example, bruises appear when bleeding occurs after an injury that does not break the skin. However, internal bleeding may not always have visible signs.

EXTERNAL BLEEDING

When bleeding occurs, the body usually responds by reducing the blood flow to the injured part. Blood vessels constrict and blood clots form at the site of the injury. This protective mechanism works

---

CONTROLLING THE BLEEDING: OPEN WOUNDS

1 Place a thick, clean compress (such as sterile gauze or a soft, clean cloth) directly over the entire wound and press firmly with your hand. Do not remove objects that are deeply embedded in the wound because this could make the bleeding worse (see page 55).

2 Continue to apply steady pressure. If blood soaks through the compress, do not remove it; add another pad over the first compress and continue applying pressure. If you are sure there is no bone fracture, a limb that is bleeding severely may be elevated above the level of the person's heart. Apply continuous direct pressure.

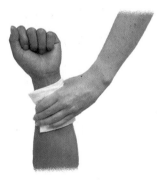

3 When the bleeding stops, apply a pressure bandage to hold the compress in place. Place the center of the bandage (gauze or cloth strips) directly over the compress. Pull steadily while wrapping the bandage around the wound. Tie a knot over the compress.

4 Check for a pulse below the level of the bandage. If there is no pulse, the bandage may be cutting off the blood supply. Loosen the bandage slightly and recheck the pulse. If the pressure needed to control the bleeding is so firm that the blood supply is cut off, loosen the bandage every 15 to 20 minutes for a minute or two.

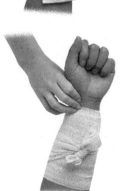

well for minor wounds and only a small amount of blood is lost. For deep wounds, this mechanism takes longer and a large amount of blood may be lost.

The amount of blood lost from a wound depends on the size of the wound and the type of vessel that has been damaged. Blood from capillaries or veins tends to flow out steadily. Blood from an artery usually spurts out. Damage to an artery is the most serious type of wound because blood is pumped out of the body at a faster rate. Prompt first aid for external bleeding is critical to prevent potentially fatal loss of blood.

Controlling bleeding

Applying direct pressure to a wound is the best way to reduce blood loss. If a wound is spurting blood, apply pressure directly over the spurting site. If this does not stop the bleeding, apply pressure at a pressure point (see USING PRESSURE POINTS on page 56). Pressure points are used in conjunction with direct pressure on the wound. Maintain pressure until the bleeding stops or medical help arrives. Never use a tourniquet to stop bleeding unless firm, direct pressure fails to control the bleeding or unless the tourniquet is necessary to control bleeding in order to save the person's life (see WARNING on page 54).

INTERNAL BLEEDING

If a person has fallen, been in an automobile accident, or had a severe blow to the body, there may be internal bleeding. Blood vessels may be damaged by a broken bone, or a damaged internal organ may be bleeding. Signs of internal bleeding are coughing up or vomiting blood; pale, cold, clammy skin; severe pain in the chest or abdomen; a swollen abdomen; or severe swelling around the injury. Abrasions or bruises on the chest, abdomen, or back should also alert you to possible internal injuries. Call for medical help immediately.

CONTROLLING THE BLEEDING: OBJECTS EMBEDDED IN A WOUND

1 Do not remove an object, such as a piece of metal or glass, or a knife, that is deeply embedded in a wound. Loose foreign material on the surface of a wound may be gently removed. To stop bleeding, apply pressure above and below an embedded object.

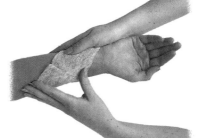

2 If you do not suspect a fracture, elevate the injured part of the body and continue applying pressure until bleeding stops. Place a piece of gauze lightly over the object and wound.

3 Put padding around the embedded object. The padding should be high enough to prevent pressure on the embedded object.

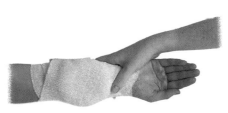

4 Use gauze or an elastic bandage to keep the padding in place. Do not wrap the bandage directly over the embedded object. Take the person to a hospital.

FIRST AID AND INFECTIOUS DISEASES

The viruses that cause acquired immune deficiency syndrome (AIDS) and some types of hepatitis can be transmitted through direct contact between the blood of an infected person and sores or open cuts on another person's skin. The risk of contracting AIDS or hepatitis by giving first aid to a bleeding person is very low but, if possible, use plastic gloves, a piece of plastic wrap, or several dressings to avoid direct contact with the person's blood.

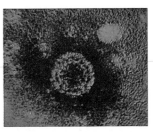

Hepatitis virus
Hepatitis is inflammation of the liver, usually caused by a virus infection. A particle of hepatitis B virus is shown above (magnified 250,000 times).

USING PRESSURE POINTS

If applying direct pressure to a wound does not stop the bleeding, you can also apply pressure at pressure points on the body. To control bleeding through the use of pressure points, press the artery that supplies blood to the wound against the underlying bone. This will decrease the flow of blood from the heart to the injured part of the body. Pressure should be applied only until bleeding stops.

Superficial temporal artery
By applying pressure on the arteries at the sides of the head, in front of the ears, you can help control bleeding from the scalp.

Facial artery
To help control bleeding from the lower part of the face, apply pressure to the notch near the angle of the lower edge of the jawbone.

Carotid artery
To help control bleeding from an artery in the neck, apply pressure to a carotid artery. (This pressure point should be used with caution in people over 60, because of the risk of causing a stroke.)

Radial artery
Bleeding from an artery in the hand may be controlled by applying pressure to the radial artery.

Brachial artery

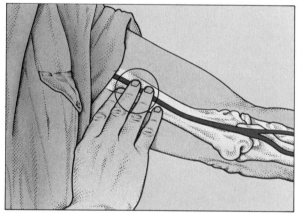

Brachial pressure point
Feel for a pulse on the inside of the person's arm. Grasp the person's arm midway between the armpit and elbow, placing your thumb on the outside of the arm and your fingers on the inside. Squeeze your fingers firmly toward your thumb against the arm bone until the bleeding stops.

Femoral artery
Pressure on the femoral artery in the center of the crease in the groin can help control bleeding from an artery in the leg.

Popliteal artery
Pressure on the popliteal artery in the back of the knee can be used to help control bleeding from an artery in the lower part of the leg.

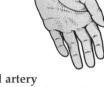

TREATING SHOCK

1 Make sure the person's airway remains open and treat the cause of shock, such as severe bleeding. Call for medical help. Keep the person lying down. Do not move the person unless necessary.

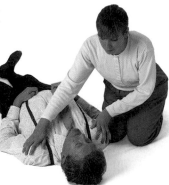

2 Unless the person has a spine, neck, or head injury, elevate the person's feet and legs. If the person has difficulty breathing, place him or her in a semireclining position. If the person vomits, place him or her on one side so vomit does not block the airway.

3 Loosen tight clothing. Keep the person comfortably warm with a coat or blanket. Do not allow the person to become overheated; overheating increases the blood flow to the vessels of the skin but diverts blood away from the body's vital organs.

4 If the person is thirsty, moisten his or her lips with water but do not give him or her anything to drink. An empty stomach is necessary because of the possible need to give the person an anesthetic at the hospital.

5 Stay with the person until medical help arrives, periodically checking his or her breathing and pulse rates. Maintain an open airway and restore breathing and circulation if necessary (see page 45).

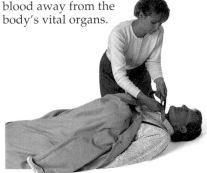

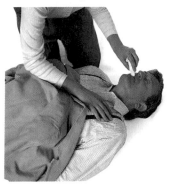

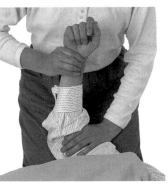

SHOCK

Shock is a condition in which the body's vital functions are threatened because not enough blood is reaching the organs and tissues. There are two main types of shock. Cardiogenic shock is caused by a failure of the heart to pump blood; hypovolemic shock is caused by a severe reduction in the volume of circulating blood. Cardiogenic shock can result from any condition that disturbs the function of the heart, such as a heart attack. Hypovolemic shock can result from severe bleeding, severe burns that cause loss of large quantities of serum (the fluid that separates from blood when it clots), or salt and water depletions caused by severe diarrhea and vomiting.

Shock that occurs with injuries can be a combination of both cardiogenic and hypovolemic shock. Giving the appropriate treatment during the first hour after a severe injury is vital to avoid the onset of shock (see above).

A person who is in shock may seem confused, restless, or anxious. The person's skin may look pale or bluish and feel cool and clammy; his or her pupils may be widely dilated. There may be trembling and weakness in the arms and legs or very slow or rapid breathing or pulse rate. Drowsiness may progress to unconsciousness, coma, and death.

Extreme pain or fear may cause psychological "shock," in which a person appears dazed, disoriented, and unable to cope with a stressful event. Another type of "shock" is a vasovagal episode, in which dizziness and fainting are caused by a reflex slowing of the heart and a drop in blood pressure. Neither of these two types of shock is life-threatening.

ANAPHYLACTIC SHOCK

Anaphylactic shock is a potentially life-threatening condition caused by an extreme allergic reaction to an insect bite or sting, a medication, or food. Seek prompt medical help. Symptoms are coughing and wheezing, difficulty breathing, severe itching or hives, severe swelling at the site of a bite or sting, stomach cramps, nausea and vomiting, dizziness, and unconsciousness.

EMERGENCY CHILDBIRTH

MOST WOMEN have some contractions during their pregnancy that are not an indication of labor. A pregnant woman never knows exactly when the first contractions of labor will begin. Ninety-eight percent of babies are delivered in a hospital. But sometimes childbirth occurs at an unexpected time or labor proceeds very quickly, and you may need to assist with the birth.

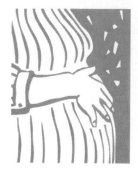

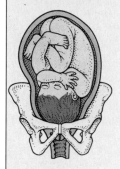

BIRTH POSITIONS

In a normal birth, the baby's head is positioned at the neck of the uterus when labor begins.

Normal birth position

A breech birth occurs when the baby is born buttocks first. A breech birth is more difficult because the baby's buttocks do not pass through the birth canal as easily as the head.

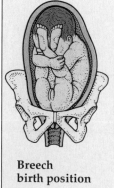

Breech birth position

If a woman is having labor contractions, call her doctor or an ambulance. Write down when the woman's contractions occur and how long they last. If you cannot get the woman to the hospital in time, follow the emergency childbirth procedures on the next page.

LABOR AND CHILDBIRTH

The delivery of a baby occurs in three stages of labor. During the first stage, the cervix (the neck of the uterus) enlarges. Cramplike pains begin in the lower part of the abdomen or the back. Contractions occur every 10 to 20 minutes. A bloody discharge from the vagina indicates that the cervix is dilating (enlarging) and the mucous plug that has blocked the cervical canal during the pregnancy has been expelled.

During the first stage of labor the membranes that surround the amniotic fluid (in which the baby floats inside the uterus) may rupture. This "water" may leak out of the vagina slowly or may be released in a gush. Once the water has broken, the baby usually begins its descent through the birth canal.

The second stage of labor begins when the cervix is fully dilated; the contractions become stronger, more frequent, and the baby is delivered. The third stage of labor is expulsion of the placenta.

PREPARING FOR EMERGENCY CHILDBIRTH

Gather the following items before the baby arrives: a clean blanket or towel to wrap the baby in, a plastic container or bag in which to place the placenta, sanitary napkins or folded cloths to be placed over the vagina after the delivery, and string or strips of cloth and sterilized scissors in case you have to tie off and cut the umbilical cord. To sterilize the scissors and string or cloth, put them in boiling water for 10 minutes. Wash your hands thoroughly with soap and water before delivering the baby.

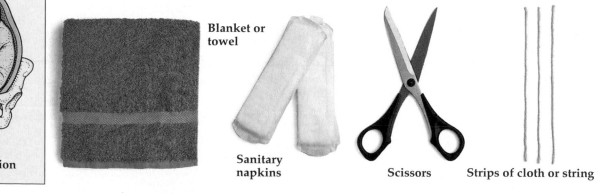

Plastic container or bag

Blanket or towel

Sanitary napkins

Scissors

Strips of cloth or string

DELIVERING THE BABY

1 Put clean sheets on a bed. If you have time, place a rubber sheet or shower curtain under the sheet to protect the mattress. Have the woman lie on her back, with knees bent, feet flat, and knees and thighs wide apart.

2 During contractions, the woman should grasp her knees, bend her head forward, hold her breath, and push downward by contracting the muscles of her diaphragm and abdomen. Try to get the woman to relax between contractions.

3 Once the baby's head emerges, guide and support the head and keep it free of blood and other secretions. If the baby's head is still inside a fluid-filled bag, carefully puncture the bag and remove any membranes from the baby's face. If the umbilical cord is wrapped around the baby's neck, gently and quickly slip the cord over the baby's head.

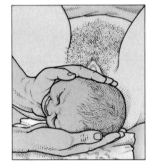

4 Continue to support the baby's head. The baby will be very slippery, so be careful. The baby will turn to the side to allow the shoulders to emerge. The upper shoulder usually emerges first; gently guide the head slightly downward. Once the upper shoulder is out, gently lift to allow the lower shoulder to emerge. Hold the baby as his or her body slides out.

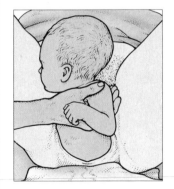

5 Gently wipe out the baby's mouth and nose. Then hold the baby with his or her head lower than the feet so secretions can drain. Support the head and body with one hand and grasp the legs and ankles with the other hand. If the baby has not cried, slap the soles of the feet or rub the baby's back. If the baby is not breathing, give artificial ventilation (see page 47).

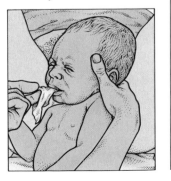

6 Once the baby starts breathing, wrap the baby, including the top and back of his or her head, in a blanket. Without pulling on the umbilical cord, place the baby on his or her side on the mother's abdomen, with the baby's head slightly lower than the rest of the body.

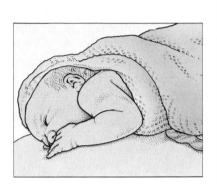

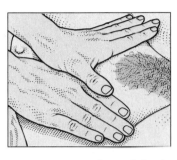

7 The placenta (also called the afterbirth) is usually delivered 5 to 20 minutes after the baby is born. To help deliver the placenta, put your hands on the mother's abdomen and gently massage her uterus (just below the navel), pressing down toward the pelvis. It is not necessary to cut the umbilical cord immediately (see below). Place sanitary napkins or clean cloths against the mother's vagina to absorb blood. Take the mother and baby to the nearest hospital emergency department as soon as possible.

CUTTING THE UMBILICAL CORD

If the mother and baby can be taken to the hospital immediately, the baby can be left attached to the umbilical cord and placenta. If you must cut the umbilical cord, follow the procedure below.

1 Tie a piece of string or strip of cloth around the cord at least 4 inches from the baby's body. Tie another piece of string 6 to 8 inches from the baby's body. Tie the strings using a tight square knot so that the circulation in the cord is cut off.

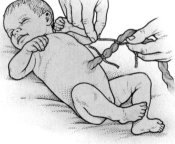

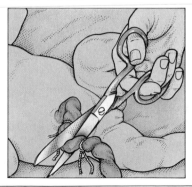

2 Cut the cord between the two pieces of string with sterilized scissors. Place the placenta in a plastic container or bag and take it with the mother and baby to the hospital so that it can be examined.

CHAPTER THREE

TYPES OF INJURIES

ONE OF THE GREATEST threats to health and life is injury. Injuries may be caused by powerful physical forces such as in a fall or an automobile accident; by environmental factors such as heat, cold, and radiation; or by chemicals such as poisons and corrosive substances. A person s age and life-style may increase his or her risk of injury. For example, injuries related to agricultural work often affect young people, who can legally work unsupervised at the age of 12. The most common causes of injuries among these young people are falls from horses or from farm buildings, kicks from horses or cows, and accidents involving farm machinery. Also, more and more children receive treatment for sports injuries every year – about 4 million are treated in hospital emergency departments and an additional 8 million are treated by their family doctor.

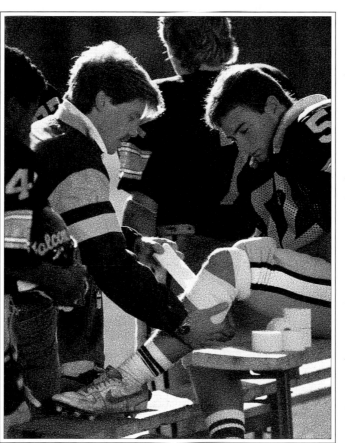

It is often easy to identify the cause and type of injury an accident victim has suffered. For example, a gash in an arm is clearly visible and you can give the appropriate first-aid treatment to the victim immediately. In other cases, the injury itself may not be visible but may cause physical signs and symptoms that you can recognize. For example, if someone has been hit in the abdomen, you might not see any obvious external signs such as bruising. However, there may be characteristic signs of internal damage, such as abdominal tenderness and tightening of the abdominal muscles when pressure is applied. Carefully evaluating the victim's condition allows you to determine the type of injury that may have occurred and to provide the appropriate first aid. Some injuries are life-threatening and require a specific type of emergency first aid. For example, artificial ventilation is essential for any injury – such as severe electric shock, some forms of poisoning, and a few types of respiratory emergencies – that causes breathing to stop.

This chapter describes a variety of injuries to different parts and systems of the body and provides guidelines for first-aid treatment. Even though our bodies have remarkable powers of recovery from injury, emergency first aid given as soon as possible after an injury helps the body recover more quickly and helps minimize any chances of permanent damage from the injury. In most cases, the injured person needs medical treatment after he or she has received prompt first aid. The first-aid treatment that you provide in the critical moments immediately after an injury may dramatically reduce the effects of the injury and may save the person's life.

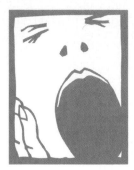

MAJOR PHYSICAL TRAUMA

T RAUMA IS THE TERM used for a strong force that causes injury; the term physical trauma refers to the resulting injury to the body's soft tissues, bones, and internal organs. Trauma is the leading cause of death among people up to age 34. More than 1 million trauma victims are hospitalized every year. The emergency first aid provided to a trauma victim during the first hour after an injury may be critical to the victim's survival.

Many minor injuries, such as bruises, scrapes, and cuts, heal rapidly without medical treatment. For injuries caused by major trauma, however, immediate intervention is usually required. At the scene of an accident where major physical trauma has occurred, the top priority of medical personnel is to save the life of the victim. Once the victim's vital functions (breathing and heartbeat) have been evaluated and resuscitation begun (if needed), the medical personnel determine the type and severity of the injuries and administer emergency first-aid treatment.

HOW DOES MAJOR TRAUMA OCCUR?

Major physical trauma occurs when a strong force is directed to the body. Two types of physical force can impact on your body. Penetrating forces (when an object is driven through the skin) cause injuries such as punctures and lacerations to internal organs. Blunt forces (when an object does not penetrate the skin) can cause internal damage to blood vessels, tissues, and organs. High-speed collisions, accidents involving heavy machinery, falls from a height, shootings, stabbings, or being struck by a flying object can cause major physical trauma.

LIFE-THREATENING PHYSICAL TRAUMA

The more severe the injury, the greater the risk to life. The location of an injury is also a critical factor in a person's survival. For example, a wound or injury that penetrates the heart may cause internal and external bleeding and interfere with the heart's ability to pump blood, resulting in almost immediate death.

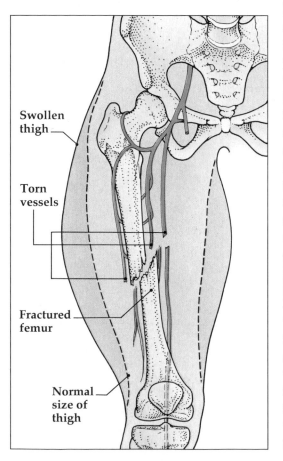

Swollen thigh

Torn vessels

Fractured femur

Normal size of thigh

Internal bleeding
Any severe blow to the body may cause internal bleeding. Internal bleeding may occur if the ends of a fractured bone damage blood vessels. Fractures of the femur (the thighbone) are often accompanied by internal bleeding, which may result in severe swelling at the site of the fractured bone.

PHYSICAL TRAUMA AND MOTOR VEHICLES

Motor-vehicle accidents can cause many types of major physical trauma. Wearing a seat belt greatly reduces your risk of injury. Passengers who are not wearing seat belts may be thrown from the vehicle. Unrestrained passengers in the front seat may be thrown against the steering wheel, dashboard, or windshield. A child sitting on an adult's lap can be crushed to death between the dashboard or windshield and the adult's body. An unrestrained passenger in the back seat may be thrown onto the people in the front seat.

Head injuries
Hitting your head on the windshield can cut your skin, injure your neck, fracture your skull or the bones in your face, or injure your brain and cause bleeding inside your skull. Shattered glass can damage your eyes and cause a loss of vision.

Chest injuries
Forceful contact with the steering wheel can cause fractures of the ribs or damage to the lungs, heart, major blood vessels, or other internal structures.

Abdominal injuries
Internal organs may be damaged in the collision, causing internal bleeding, rupture of hollow internal organs (such as the intestines), or fractures of the spine or pelvic bones.

Arm injuries
Fractures of bones in your wrist and arms and lacerations of the skin are often the result of bracing yourself for the impact of the collision or covering your face with your hands.

Leg injuries
Impact with the steering wheel column can cause multiple fractures and lacerations of the legs. If the body of the vehicle is pushed inward onto the driver, his or her legs may be crushed.

Neck and spinal injuries

A trauma victim with serious head or facial injuries may also have injuries to the part of the spine in the neck. To prevent damage to the spinal cord, the victim should not be moved until medical help arrives unless absolutely necessary (see page 73). If the spinal cord is damaged, the victim may have temporary or permanent paralysis (loss of movement). Medical personnel will evaluate the victim's general condition and assess the ABCs (airway, breathing, and circulation) of the victim's vital functions (see page 45). They will administer the first aid needed for any injuries and then immobilize the victim on a backboard for transportation to the hospital.

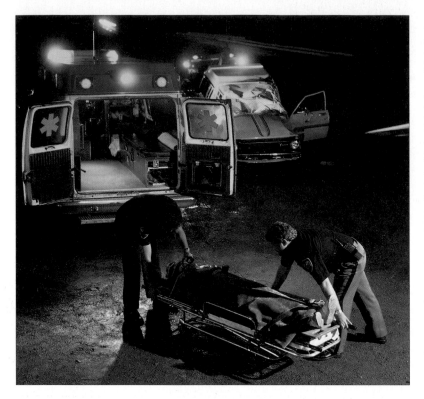

Call an ambulance
While first aid provided by a bystander can make the difference between life and death in the first few minutes after an accident, prompt treatment by medical professionals is essential for major physical trauma.

SEVERED LIMB

If a person's limb has been severed, always treat the person first – the severed limb should be a second-ary concern. In some cases, an amputated part can be reattached. After you stabilize the person's condition, wrap the ampu-tated part in a moist clean cloth and put it in a plastic bag. Put the bag in ice water and take it with you to the hospital emergency department.

BLEEDING

An injury that causes severe bleeding, such as amputation of a body part (see box below left) or a deep laceration that severs an artery, can cause death quickly if the bleeding is not stopped.

Blunt trauma may cause internal and external bleeding as a result of damage to internal structures. Injuries that penetrate the skin and damage blood vessels cause external bleeding. Controlling bleeding (see pages 54 and 55) and treating the victim for shock (see page 57) are critical before medical help arrives. If necessary, medical personnel will start intravenous administration of fluids.

BREATHING PROBLEMS

A blow to the head may interfere with the body's process of respiration, causing breathing to stop. Without immediate airway control (see OPENING THE AIRWAY on page 46) or artificial ventilation (see page 47), brain damage or death can occur within 4 to 6 minutes.

A chest injury may also lead to breathing difficulties. In victims with breathing prob-lems caused by a punctured lung (see below), medical personnel check the ABCs of the victim's vital functions (see page 45). Oxygen and fluids are admin-istered. The medical personnel attach pads for a heart rate monitor to the victim's chest. Then they listen to the lungs to check breath sounds and to rule out a pneumothorax (see page 80). If necessary, a needle may be inserted through the chest wall to relieve pres-sure. The medical personnel then trans-port the victim to the nearest appropri-ate hospital emergency department.

FIRST AID FOR MAJOR PHYSICAL TRAUMA

If you are the first person at the scene of an accident and are trained in first aid, first make sure that it is safe for you to approach. Treat the victims who may have life-threatening injuries immedi-ately, using the ABCs of emergency first aid (see page 45). Phone 911 (or your local emergency number) as soon as pos-sible. While you wait for medical help, provide first aid for all other victims. Obtaining information on how the acci-dent happened from witnesses or vic-tims may also be very useful to the emer-gency services team.

Punctured lung
The ends of a fractured rib can puncture a lung and cause breathing difficulties.

Collapsed lung

CASE HISTORY
A TIRED DRIVER

Tom had been working late at his drawing board, finishing the design for a brochure he needed to present to his boss first thing the next morning. He left the office after midnight. Exhausted, he got into his car and started home, completely forgetting to fasten his seat belt.

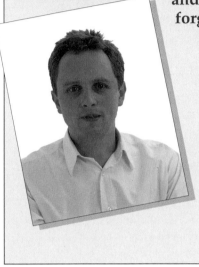

PERSONAL DETAILS
Name Tom Carlson
Age 35
Occupation Graphic designer
Family Both parents died in an airplane crash when Tom was 8 years old.

THE INCIDENT

Tom drives off on his usual route home. As he struggles to stay awake, his car drifts off the road and smashes into a telephone pole. The impact of the crash propels Tom forward and over the steering wheel and into the windshield.

FIRST AID

A passing motorist sees the accident and pulls off the road to see if he can be of any assistance. He sees Tom is badly injured and calls for an ambulance. The paramedics arrive to find Tom slumped over the steering wheel. He is breathing but unconscious. Tom is bleeding severely from deep cuts on his scalp and on his right arm. The paramedics administer the necessary first aid to control the bleeding and then find that his left ankle is broken. They immobilize his broken ankle as well as his neck and back (in case he has a spinal injury) before moving him out of the car and onto a stretcher. On the way to the hospital, the paramedics continue direct pressure to his cuts and insert an intravenous line to begin replacement of fluids to prevent shock. Tom regains consciousness in the ambulance. He tells the paramedics he must have fallen asleep at the wheel because he doesn't remember hitting the telephone pole.

AT THE HOSPITAL

In the emergency department, oxygen is given and intravenous fluids are continuously administered while the doctors thoroughly evaluate Tom's condition. The cuts on his scalp and right arm are stitched closed. Because of his head injury and loss of consciousness a computed tomography (CT) scan of Tom's head is done; the scan shows no bleeding inside his skull. Blood tests and X-rays are performed. Although Tom's chest is severely bruised, X-rays do not show any broken ribs or injury to his lungs or heart. The X rays confirm the ankle fracture, which will require surgery. A metal plate and screws are used to realign and immobilize the broken bones.

THE OUTCOME

After surgery, Tom stays in the hospital for several days. At a follow-up visit with the surgeon a week later, the doctor tells Tom that the bones in his ankle are healing well. He tells Tom that the injured muscles in his right arm will become stronger as they continue to heal, but he may not have the strength in that arm that he had before the accident.

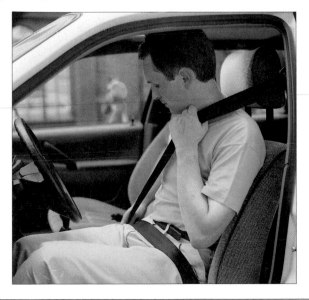

Driving safely
After his accident, Tom vows that he will never again drive when he is tired and will always wear a seat belt, even if driving only a few blocks.

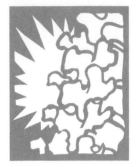

FRACTURES AND BACK INJURIES

A FRACTURE IS THE TERM used to describe a crack or complete break in a bone. In most cases, a broken bone is not life-threatening. Bone fractures are a serious threat only when blood vessels, nerve tissue such as the spinal cord, or vital organs such as the heart or lungs are damaged by the ends of a fractured bone.

A strong force is usually required to break a healthy bone. The way a bone fractures depends on the type of force that is applied to the bone and on the person's age. Cartilage makes up part of a child's bones and is softer and much less brittle than the hardened tissue found in mature bone. Children's bones tend to bend or splinter rather than break under stress; bones become brittle and break more easily as we get older.

WHAT CAUSES A FRACTURE?

A bone may break at any point where a strong force is applied; a bone may also break at a point some distance from the force. For example, if a fall results in force being transmitted along the length of the arm bones, the full force of the fall is placed on the collarbone and it can break. A fracture may also occur when a muscle pulls too violently on a bone.

Symptoms of a fracture

In some cases, you can hear a snapping sound when a bone fractures. The site of a fracture is painful and may be swollen and have a bluish coloration caused by internal bleeding. It may be difficult or impossible to move the injured part. A grating sensation may be felt as the ends of the fractured bone rub together. The injured part may also move in an abnormal way or appear deformed.

In some severe breaks, the ends of a broken bone protrude through the skin. This is called an open fracture. A person with an open fracture may require treatment for bleeding and shock (see page 54).

TREATING FRACTURES

Any of the 206 bones that make up the human skeleton can fracture. Arm fractures occur frequently in all age groups and are usually caused by falls. The most common sites of broken bones are in the hands and feet.

Finger and toe fractures

X-rays are usually necessary to determine whether bones in the fingers and toes have been broken. First-aid treatment of a fractured finger or toe may involve simply strapping the injured

Wrist fractures
Falling onto an outstretched hand may fracture a bone in the wrist. Some fractures cause misalignment (see below). In the emergency department, fractured bones may be manipulated back into position and a cast applied. Surgery may be required. If you injure your wrist, hand, or fingers, remove your rings on that hand because, if your fingers swell, the rings can restrict the circulation.

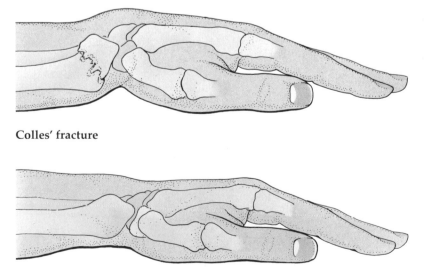

Colles' fracture

Normal wrist

TYPES OF FRACTURES

Long bones (such as the bones in the legs) are very strong and can resist many forces applied along the length of the bone. However, long bones are much more likely to break if a strong force is applied across the bone. Fractures most often occur at the narrowest point of a bone, where the bone is weakest. The type of fracture depends on the nature of the force applied to the bone.

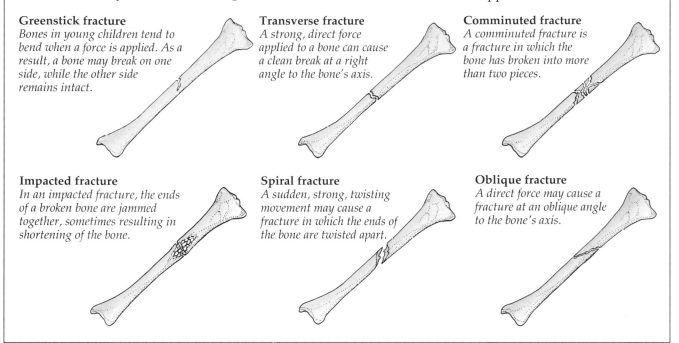

Greenstick fracture
Bones in young children tend to bend when a force is applied. As a result, a bone may break on one side, while the other side remains intact.

Transverse fracture
A strong, direct force applied to a bone can cause a clean break at a right angle to the bone's axis.

Comminuted fracture
A comminuted fracture is a fracture in which the bone has broken into more than two pieces.

Impacted fracture
In an impacted fracture, the ends of a broken bone are jammed together, sometimes resulting in shortening of the bone.

Spiral fracture
A sudden, strong, twisting movement may cause a fracture in which the ends of the bone are twisted apart.

Oblique fracture
A direct force may cause a fracture at an oblique angle to the bone's axis.

finger or toe to an adjacent digit with tape and gauze to splint and immobilize the fractured bone (see page 86). Because of the coordination required in the hand, fractures of bones in the fingers may require physical therapy after the fracture heals. Elevation of a fractured finger or toe may help reduce swelling.

Leg fractures

Fractures of the ankle and lower part of the leg are common sports injuries. Strapping the injured leg to the uninjured leg immobilizes the fractured bone and may reduce the pain; take the person to the nearest hospital emergency department.

Fracture of the hip

Hip fractures often occur as the result of a fall, particularly in women who are past the menopause. A person who may have a hip fracture should not be moved until medical help arrives. Do not give the person anything to eat or drink be-fore medical help arrives, because he or she may require anesthesia if surgery is needed to repair the fractured bone.

BACK INJURIES

Any injury of the spine can damage the spinal cord, causing numbness, muscle weakness, or paralysis (loss of move-ment). A person with a suspected spinal injury should never be moved unless the neck and back are completely immobi-lized (see page 69). Improperly moving a person who has a spinal injury can worsen damage to the spinal cord.

A fracture or dislocation of the verte-brae in the spine may be caused by any force that crushes vertebrae together or causes sudden, extreme bending of the spine. In severe dislocations and frac-tures, the vertebrae may crush or sever the spinal cord. Swelling caused by a severely fractured or dislocated vertebra may press on and injure the spinal cord.

WARNING

A plaster or plastic cast applied to immobilize a fracture is too tight if the cast causes severe pain and additional swelling or the injured limb feels numb or cold and appears blue. A cast that is too tight must be loos-ened or removed and replaced. Call your doctor or go to the nearest hospital emergency department.

SPLINTING AND IMMOBILIZING FRACTURES AND BACK INJURIES

Moving a limb that has a broken bone can cause severe pain and more damage to the bone or to the soft tissues (such as blood vessels and nerves) near the bone. Always apply a splint to immobilize a limb that might be fractured before moving the person. A splint can be made from objects such as boards, sticks or branches, or several rolled newspapers. To ensure a broken bone is completely immobilized, a splint should extend beyond the joint above and the joint below the fracture. Do not move a person with a suspected spinal injury unless he or she is in immediate danger. Wait for medical help to arrive.

INJURY TO THE WRIST AND LOWER PART OF THE ARM

1 Place the injured arm at a right angle across the person's chest, with the palm facing inward. Apply a padded splint on both sides of the arm. The splint can be made of several folded newspapers and should reach from the elbow to well beyond the wrist.

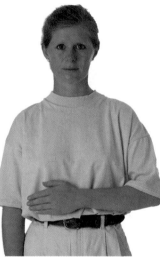

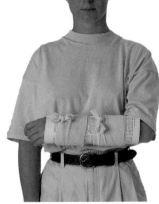

2 Tie the splint in place above and below the fracture.

3 Support the arm with a wide sling that elevates the fingers 3 or 4 inches above the level of the elbow. Elevation of the lower part of the arm in this way reduces the amount of swelling. Take the person to the nearest hospital emergency department.

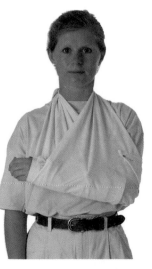

FRACTURES OF THE LOWER PART OF THE LEG

1 If necessary, carefully and slowly straighten the injured leg, supporting the leg above and below the fracture. Place padding, such as a folded blanket or coat, between the person's legs and carefully move the legs together.

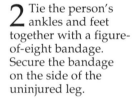

2 Tie the person's ankles and feet together with a figure-of-eight bandage. Secure the bandage on the side of the uninjured leg.

3 Tie the legs together in two or three places, including just above and below the knees. Tie all knots on the side of the uninjured leg. Wait for medical help to arrive.

BACK INJURIES

A person with a suspected spinal injury should never be moved unless he or she is in a life-threatening situation; wait for medical help to arrive. Improperly moving a person who has a spinal injury can damage the spinal cord more severely. If the person must be moved, the neck and back must always be completely immobilized first.

1 Place a long, wide board beside the person. Keeping the person's head, neck, and back in alignment, gently roll the person onto his or her side.

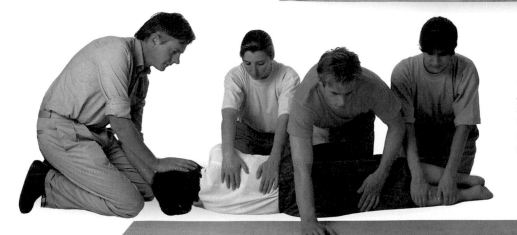

2 Pull the board toward the person and gently roll him or her onto the board. If the person is vomiting, he or she should be lying on one side to prevent choking.

3 Tie the person to the board in several places (but not tight enough to restrict breathing). Make sure that his or her head cannot move in any direction. Carefully move the person to safety.

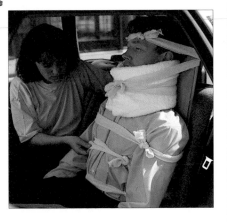

Use of a short back board
If a person must be moved from a vehicle, a short board should be used to immobilize his or her back and neck. Slide the board down behind the person and tie it securely to the person's head, neck, and chest (but not tight enough to restrict breathing). With the board in place, carefully lift the person from the vehicle.

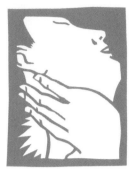

HEAD AND NECK INJURIES

EVERY YEAR, 10 million people suffer head injuries. Head and neck injuries may damage the brain or spinal cord. Medical personnel should always be called to treat accident victims with possible head or neck injuries, even if there are no obvious signs of internal damage. Always assume that anyone found unconscious after an accident has a major injury to the brain or spinal cord.

Bleeding in the skull
Bleeding may occur between the inner surface of the skull and the tough membrane called the dura mater (epidural hemorrhage), under the dura mater (subdural hemorrhage), between the arachnoid membrane and the surface of the brain (subarachnoid hemorrhage), and deep in the brain itself (intracerebral hemorrhage).

Subarachnoid hemorrhage

Dura mater

Subdural hemorrhage

Epidural hemorrhage

Intracerebral hemorrhage

Bleeding in the brain
Bleeding deep inside the brain is called an intracerebral hemorrhage.

A head injury that causes bleeding inside the skull is a serious threat to the brain. A fracture or dislocation of the vertebrae in the neck can injure the spinal cord, which can cause paralysis (loss of movement) below the level of the injury.

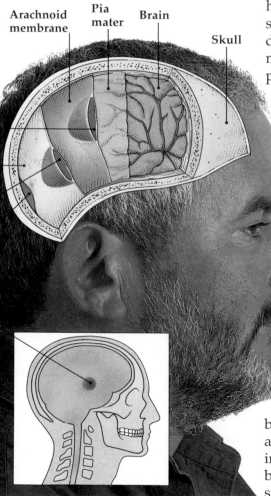

Arachnoid membrane **Pia mater** **Brain**

Skull

HEAD INJURIES

Head injuries occur in about two thirds of people who are injured in motor-vehicle accidents. When traveling in a vehicle, the body of the driver or passenger has a momentum proportional to the speed of movement. If the vehicle suddenly decelerates, the body continues to move at the original speed, causing powerful strain on the neck.

Falling onto the head from a height (such as diving into shallow water and hitting your head on the bottom) and striking the head against a hard object are two common causes of head injuries. Bullet wounds and direct blows to the head with sharp or blunt instruments also cause serious – and often fatal – head injuries.

Skull fractures

Fractures of the skull may cause damage to the brain and internal bleeding (see left). Fractures of the base of the skull sometimes cause bleeding from the ear. These fractures may also cause cerebrospinal fluid (the fluid that cushions the brain) to leak out from inside the skull and open a pathway for bacteria to cause infection. If a skull fracture results in bone fragments being pushed inward, surgery may be required.

FIRST AID FOR HEAD INJURIES

Check the person to see if he or she is breathing. If the person is not breathing, start artificial ventilation (see page 47). Do not twist or rotate the head. Cover any head wounds with a clean bandage.

1 Use a clean triangular bandage and put the center of the base of the bandage across the person's forehead, just above the eyes, with the point of the bandage at the back of the head.

2 Take the two long ends of the bandage and cross them over, just below the back of the head.

3 Bring the ends of the bandage around to the front of the head and tie the ends together.

4 Tuck in the point of the bandage at the back of the neck where the points were crossed over.

Internal bleeding

A head injury that causes a person to become unconscious, recover consciousness, and then lapse back into unconsciousness is potentially dangerous. Take the person to the hospital immediately; these signs may indicate bleeding inside the skull, which can be fatal. An enlarging hematoma (a swelling containing blood) in the skull compresses the brain and may push the brain downward, forcing the brain stem into the small spinal canal, usually causing death.

Concussion

A concussion is a head injury caused by sudden movement of the brain within the skull, which may result in a temporary disordered state of consciousness (see right). This type of head injury frequently occurs after collisions in contact sports such as football and hockey.

NECK INJURIES

Neck injuries may result from motor-vehicle accidents, sports activities, and falls. Serious neck injuries may be caused by a direct blow to the neck or a sudden, forceful bending of the neck, either forward or backward, that fractures vertebrae in the neck and damages the spinal cord (see BROKEN NECK on page 72).

FIRST AID FOR CONCUSSION

The signs and symptoms of a concussion vary, depending on the severity of the injury. A mild concussion may cause temporary loss of memory of recent events, dizziness, and ringing in the ears, but no loss of consciousness or coordination. A more severe concussion causes loss of consciousness that may last from a few seconds to longer than 5 minutes. A person with a head injury who has lost consciousness needs immediate medical attention.

1 Check whether the person is breathing (see page 45) and has a pulse (see page 49). Call for medical help.

2 Do not move the person because this may worsen a possible spinal injury. Test the person's level of responsiveness by pinching the skin on the back of his or her hand to see if he or she responds to pain.

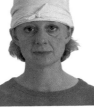

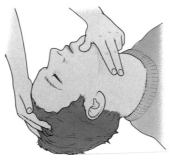

Skull

Bleeding

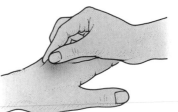

3 If unconsciousness persists, the person may have increased pressure inside the skull, a serious condition in which blood accumulates in the skull and puts pressure on the brain.

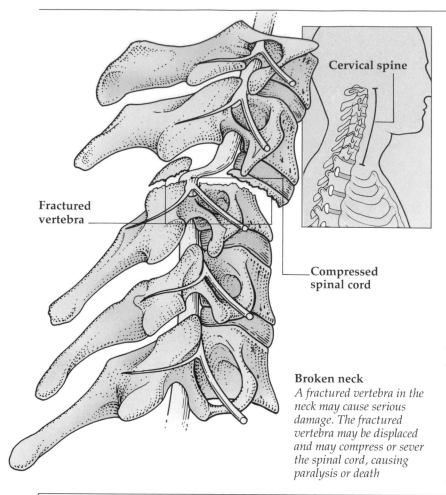

Cervical spine

Fractured vertebra

Compressed spinal cord

Broken neck
A fractured vertebra in the neck may cause serious damage. The fractured vertebra may be displaced and may compress or sever the spinal cord, causing paralysis or death

A common neck injury from motor-vehicle accidents is a whiplash, caused by a sudden, sharp whipping movement of the neck. Muscles and ligaments may be strained or sprained. Properly positioned headrests help minimize the severity of whiplash injuries (see page 38).

Damage to the spinal cord

The spinal cord contains all the nerve tracts that connect the brain with the rest of the body. The spinal cord is protected by the vertebrae, which form a bony canal that runs down the length of the spine. With sufficient force, the nerve fibers of the spinal cord may be severely compressed or severed, cutting off communications between the nerves in the body below the level of the injury and the brain. As a result, paralysis (loss of movement) and loss of sensation and control of the bladder and bowels may occur. Also, the body's vital organs may be unable to function, causing death. Severed nerve fibers in the spinal cord cannot regenerate and the effects are permanent.

SIGNS AND SYMPTOMS OF HEAD AND NECK INJURIES

Look for the following signs and symptoms when evaluating an accident victim for the possibility of a head or neck injury. You should always suspect a neck injury if the victim has a head injury.

HEAD INJURY
◆ A cut in the scalp, a lump or a bruise on the scalp, or a depression in the contour of the skull. A bone depression is often hidden by swelling of the scalp.
◆ Drowsiness, confusion, difficulty speaking, or unconsciousness.
◆ Vomiting or seizures.
◆ Blood or clear fluid leaking from the nose, mouth, or (especially) the ear.
◆ A headache.
◆ A pale or flushed face.
◆ Slow or irregular pulse.
◆ Different-sized pupils of the eyes.

NECK INJURY
◆ A headache.
◆ Stiff neck.
◆ Inability of the victim to move.
◆ A tingling "pins-and-needles" feeling in any part of the body, especially in the arms or legs.
◆ Loss of voluntary movement of any part of the body.

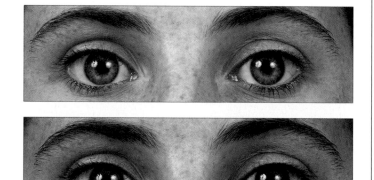

Changes in pupil size
In the top illustration, the pupils are fairly small and normal. In the lower illustration, the pupils are unequal in size and may indicate the victim has a head injury. Call for medical help immediately.

MOVING A PERSON WITH A SUSPECTED NECK INJURY

Never move a person with a possible neck injury unless you have trained medical assistance. Any movement could injure or worsen damage to the spinal cord and cause paralysis or death. Call for medical help immediately. However, if the person is in danger and must be moved, he or she must be moved on a board, with the head, neck, and torso completely immobilized. Three or four people are needed to move the victim.

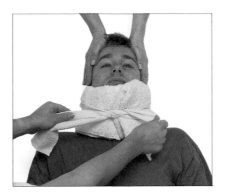

1 Fold a towel to the width of about 4 inches and carefully slide the towel under the person's neck. DO NOT MOVE THE PERSON'S HEAD OR NECK IN ANY WAY. Carefully and firmly secure the towel, but not so tightly that it obstructs breathing.

2 Working in unison, keep the person's head, neck, and torso completely immobilized and roll the person slightly onto his or her side. Slide the board under the person's body, and then roll the person back onto the board.

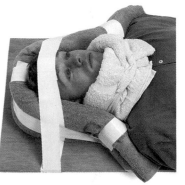

3 Fold and tape another towel to the width of 4 inches and wrap the towel around the top of the person's head. To prevent movement, secure the person's head to the board by taping across his or her forehead.

WHAT YOU NEED

◆ A wide board (such as a door) that reaches from above the head down to the feet
◆ Towels
◆ Tape and strips of strong cloth
◆ Three or four people to help move the person

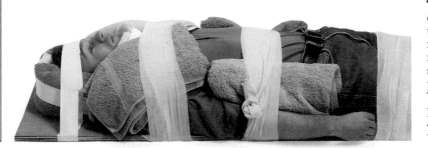

4 Place folded towels, clothing, or blankets around the person's head, neck, and sides to make an informal splint that will prevent movement. Tie or tape the person to the board, across the chest, waist, and legs.

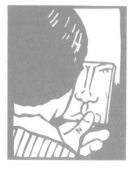

FACIAL INJURIES

ALTHOUGH FACIAL INJURIES usually require prompt medical treatment, in most cases they are not life-threatening. Injuries to the face are often caused by automobile accidents, collisions during sports activities, falls, fires, and assault. Injuries to the eyes are frequently caused by tools. You can help prevent eye or other facial injuries by always using the proper safety equipment when you are working with tools around your house or at your job.

Facial injuries vary in severity from a simple nosebleed to severe wounds and fractures of the bones of the face. Breathing difficulties may occur if displaced jaw or facial bones or excessive bleeding into the mouth and throat cause obstruction of the airway. For severe facial injuries, immediate first aid is essential to make sure that the person's airway is open and to control bleeding. First-aid treatment of some less severe types of facial injuries is described below.

NOSEBLEEDS

The many blood vessels in the nose lie close to the surface of the nasal lining. Bleeding from the nose may be caused by any sort of damage to the nose, such as forcefully blowing your nose or scratching the inside of your nose. In most cases, a nosebleed is not serious and the bleeding is easily controlled (see below left). If the bleeding does not stop with firm, direct pressure on both nostrils, call your doctor. Your doctor may pack the nasal cavities with gauze or cauterize the damaged blood vessel (that is, use a medical instrument or a chemical to stop the bleeding). If a nosebleed or a leakage of thin fluid from your nose begins after a head injury, there may be a fracture of the base of the skull; get to a hospital immediately.

TONGUE AND LIP INJURIES

The tongue and lips bleed heavily if cut or deeply bitten. To control bleeding from a wound on your tongue or lips, apply constant, direct pressure. To help grip your tongue, place a piece of gauze between your forefinger and thumb and firmly squeeze the edges of the cut together. See a doctor immediately.

Broken nose
A strong physical force hitting your nose can fracture or displace bones and cartilage in the nose (see X-ray at right). The bones and cartilage may need to be realigned after the swelling has subsided. The doctor will give you a local anesthetic and then manipulate the bones and cartilage back into place.

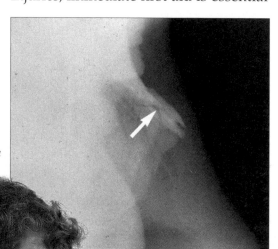

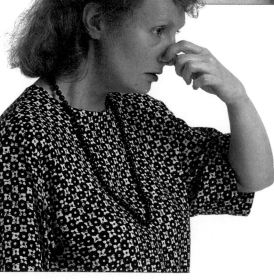

Stopping a nosebleed
Most nosebleeds can be stopped by pinching the nostrils together for about 15 minutes. Sit down and lower your chin slightly toward your chest. Breathe with your mouth open so that blood clots do not obstruct your airway. Apply a cold pack on your nose or face to help constrict the blood vessels.

FIRST AID FOR A BROKEN JAW

A broken jaw may result from automobile accidents, collisions in contact sports, or a blow from a fist to the jaw. A broken jaw causes pain, tenderness, and swelling. There may be numbness on one side of the face, and the mouth may not close completely. The muscles that move the lower jaw may pull the fractured part of the jawbone out of alignment. Breathing difficulties can occur if the airway becomes obstructed. A broken jaw must be immobilized until it can be treated by a doctor. If a neck injury is suspected, also immobilize the person's neck.

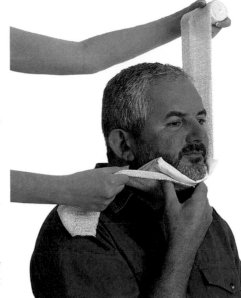

1 Call for medical help. Put a pad of soft cloth or a folded towel beneath the chin. Place a strip of cloth or a bandage under the chin while the person holds the pad to his or her jaw.

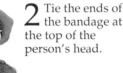

2 Tie the ends of the bandage at the top of the person's head.

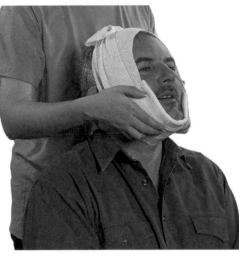

3 If the person has difficulty breathing, gently pull the jaw forward and hold the jaw in that position until medical help arrives. If bleeding or excessive secretion of saliva occurs, use a piece of gauze or clean cloth to soak the fluids from the person's mouth.

DENTAL INJURIES

Injuries that fracture the bones in the jaw may also damage teeth. Chipped or broken teeth can be crowned, bonded (by applying a synthetic material to the tooth surface), or reshaped. If a tooth has been loosened and is partially out of its socket, press the tooth back into place and call your dentist immediately. If a tooth has been knocked out, apply direct pressure to the empty socket to control bleeding. Save the tooth (see right), and call your dentist immediately. Your dentist can often replace the tooth in the socket and temporarily immobilize the tooth with a wire or plastic splint.

Injuries to the soft tissues in your mouth can be caused by common products. Excessive use of mouthwash (several times a day) can kill the harmless bacteria in your mouth, resulting in growth of harmful bacteria that may cause ulceration or infection. Stop using any product that irritates the inside of your mouth and call your dentist. Also, never place an aspirin alongside an aching tooth; the aspirin can cause a chemical burn to your cheek and gums.

Saving a knocked-out tooth
If a tooth has been knocked out, keep the tooth in your mouth or soak it in milk to keep the tooth alive.

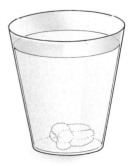

EYE INJURIES

Common causes of eye injury include a foreign object in the eye, chemicals that burn the eye, and a hard, direct blow to the eye. Any of these causes of injury can be very serious because vision may be permanently impaired. Call your ophthalmologist (eye doctor) immediately after any eye injury.

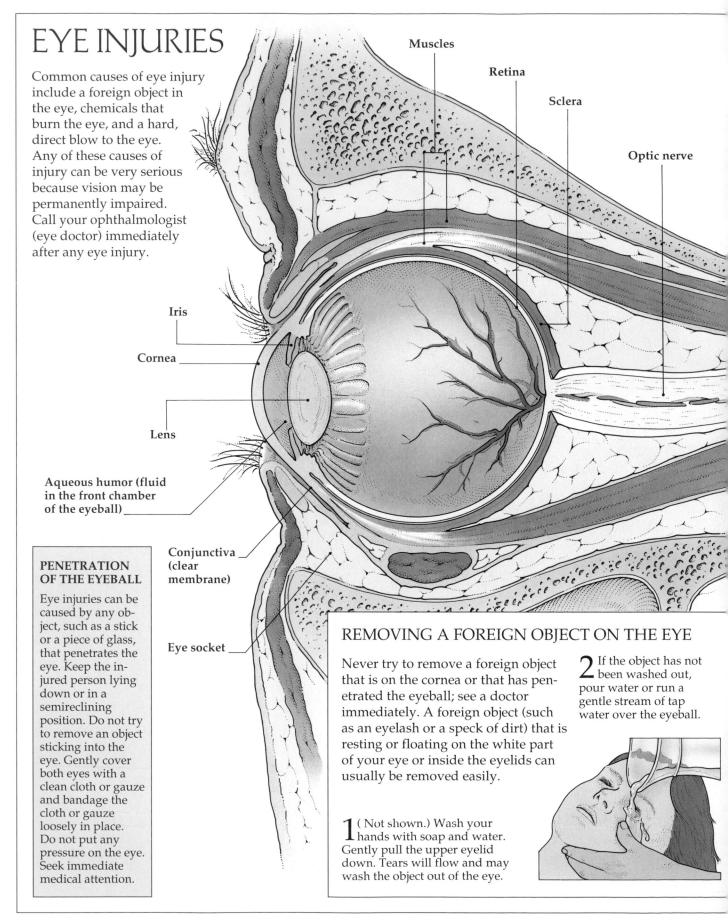

Muscles

Retina

Sclera

Optic nerve

Iris

Cornea

Lens

Aqueous humor (fluid in the front chamber of the eyeball)

Conjunctiva (clear membrane)

Eye socket

PENETRATION OF THE EYEBALL

Eye injuries can be caused by any object, such as a stick or a piece of glass, that penetrates the eye. Keep the injured person lying down or in a semireclining position. Do not try to remove an object sticking into the eye. Gently cover both eyes with a clean cloth or gauze and bandage the cloth or gauze loosely in place. Do not put any pressure on the eye. Seek immediate medical attention.

REMOVING A FOREIGN OBJECT ON THE EYE

Never try to remove a foreign object that is on the cornea or that has penetrated the eyeball; see a doctor immediately. A foreign object (such as an eyelash or a speck of dirt) that is resting or floating on the white part of your eye or inside the eyelids can usually be removed easily.

2 If the object has not been washed out, pour water or run a gentle stream of tap water over the eyeball.

1 (Not shown.) Wash your hands with soap and water. Gently pull the upper eyelid down. Tears will flow and may wash the object out of the eye.

Black eye

A black eye is a common result of an injury to the eye area or the forehead. The discoloration is caused by blood leaking into the skin tissues around the eyes. Apply cold compresses to the injured area and seek prompt medical attention. The blood that has collected in the tissues around the eye will gradually be reabsorbed in about 2 to 3 weeks as the blood is broken down by enzymes.

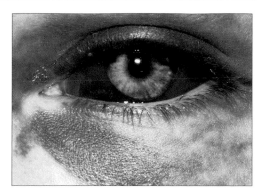

Chemical burns to the eyes

Chemicals such as drain openers and bleaches can damage the eyes permanently. Immediately flush the eye with running water for at least 10 minutes; the eyelids should be held open. Make sure the water flushes out all parts of the eyes. Cover the eyes with gauze and bandage the gauze in place. Get medical help immediately.

Subconjunctival hemorrhage

A subconjunctival hemorrhage (bleeding under the conjunctiva – the white of the eye) causes a layer of blood to form in the conjunctiva. This condition is usually caused by a minor injury that breaks blood vessels. The blood is usually reabsorbed slowly on its own. If this condition is the result of a blow to the eye, see your ophthalmologist.

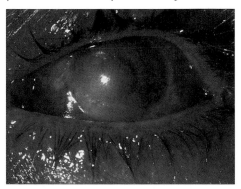

Hyphema

Hyphema is bleeding inside the front of the eye, often caused by a direct injury to the eye. The blood originates in the damaged iris or the muscle that focuses the iris and enters the fluid in the front part of the eye. Most hyphemas are absorbed in a few days, but they can be associated with serious eye damage and recurrent bleeding; seek medical attention as soon as possible.

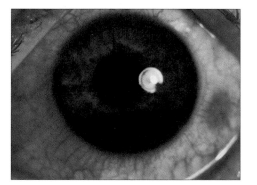

RUPTURED SCLERA

Call your ophthalmologist immediately if you experience a blow to the eye. Rupture of the sclera (the white outer covering of the eye) is one of the most serious consequences of such an injury. The risk of permanent loss of vision or loss of the eye is high if the sclera has ruptured. Surgery may be necessary.

3 If this is unsuccessful, pull down the lower eyelid. If the object is visible, carefully remove it with a moistened, clean tissue or cloth.

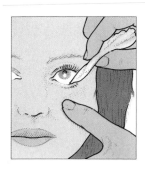

4 If the particle is not visible, pull the lashes of the upper eyelid down, with the eye looking down. Place a cotton-tipped swab across the eyelid and pull the eyelid back over the swab. If the object is visible, gently remove it with a moistened, clean tissue or cloth.

Blow-out fracture

A hard blow to the eye may cause a sudden rise in pressure inside the eye socket that can fracture the floor of the socket, causing the eyeball to sink. You may experience double vision if the injury damages the eye muscles. See your ophthalmologist immediately.

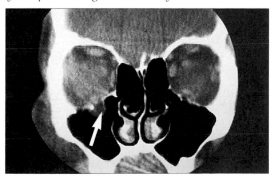

CASE HISTORY
A RUSHED FIX-IT JOB

ONE SATURDAY, **Henry was putting his golf clubs in the trunk of his car when his youngest son came into the garage and asked him to fix his model car. Henry saw that a jagged piece of metal was preventing one of the wheels from turning. Concerned that his son might cut himself on the piece of metal, Henry decided to grind down the sharp edge in his workshop.**

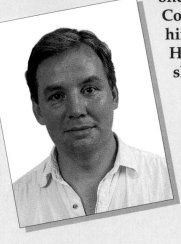

PERSONAL DETAILS
Name Henry Gallery
Age 44
Occupation Computer software salesman
Family Married, with three children.

THE INCIDENT

Henry's power grinder is right on the workbench in his garage, and he knows it should only take a couple of minutes to fix his son's model car. His safety goggles are not hanging in the usual place. Henry is in a hurry to get to the golf course and doesn't want to look for the goggles, so he starts using the power grinder without them. Suddenly, a small fragment of metal flies off the model car and hits him in his right eye.

FIRST AID

Henry's son runs into the house to get his mother. Henry's wife rushes into the garage and sees him leaning over the workbench, with his hand over his right eye. She sends her son to get the first-aid kit. Henry is in a lot of pain and is unable to open his right eye. Henry's wife gently places a piece of gauze over his right eye and puts a loose bandage over both eyes. She drives him to the ophthalmologist's office.

AT THE DOCTOR'S OFFICE

Henry tells the ophthalmologist what happened. The ophthalmologist places a drop of a local anesthetic in Henry's eye and then examines the injured eye using a slit-lamp microscope (see below). A small fragment of steel lies near the center of the cornea. The ophthalmologist lifts out the metal fragment. Although there is no sign of metal farther inside the eye, the ophthalmologist tells Henry to go to the hospital emergency department for an X-ray. He gives Henry an antibiotic to prevent infection and places atropine drops in Henry's eye to dilate the pupil and prevent an increase of pressure in the eye. The ophthalmologist applies a sterile pad and asks Henry to make an appointment to come back in 2 days.

THE OUTCOME

At the follow-up appointment, the doctor notes that the cornea is healing and that the vision in Henry's right eye has improved but is still cloudy. He tells Henry that the injury will leave only a small scar but he will have some loss of the vision in his right eye. The injury could have been more serious if the fragment had penetrated deeper into the eye, possibly causing blindness. Henry always wears goggles now when he works with tools.

Examining the injured eye
The ophthalmologist uses a slit-lamp microscope to examine Henry's injured eye. The doctor finds a small fragment of metal and gently removes it.

WARNING

Never poke anything, such as cotton swabs, paper clips, matches, or pencils, into your ear. The object may break off in the ear canal and be difficult to remove. Poking an object into your ear may also rupture the eardrum and cause infection of the middle ear.

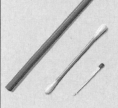

A ruptured eardrum
An eardrum can be ruptured by poking objects into the ear, by a serious head injury, by a loud, nearby explosion, or by infection of the middle ear. Symptoms of a ruptured eardrum are bleeding from inside the ear, pain, and hearing loss. Call your doctor if you suspect you have a ruptured eardrum.

Ruptured eardrum

EAR INJURIES

Injuries to the outer ear may cause severe bleeding but are usually not life-threatening. Blood or a clear, thin fluid running out of the ear canal may indicate a serious head injury; call an ambulance. Bleeding from the ear may also be caused by a ruptured eardrum (see below). Do not put anything into the ear canal to absorb the blood. Turn the person's head so that the blood can drain out (but only if a neck injury is not suspected), cover the ear with a clean cloth, and get medical help immediately.

Outer ear injuries
The outer ear (called the pinna) can be torn, cut, or partially severed. Cover the wound with sterile gauze, apply direct pressure on the wound to control bleeding, bandage the ear to keep the gauze in place, and take the person to a doctor immediately.

Removing an insect from the ear
Tilt the head so that the affected ear is on top. Trickle warm water or oil (baby, mineral, or olive oil) into the ear to immobilize the insect. See your doctor so he or she can remove the insect.

Foreign objects in the ear
Children often put small items, such as beans, stones, or beads, in their ears. Do not put water or oil in the ear to flush out the object; this can cause some objects to swell. If the obstruction (such as a piece of paper or cotton) is clearly visible and can be grasped easily, hold the child's head completely still and remove the object with tweezers. See your doctor as soon as possible to make sure all of the object has been removed. Do not try to remove the blockage if you cannot grasp it easily; you may push the object farther into the ear. Take the child to the emergency department immediately.

If an insect enters the ear canal and is alive and buzzing, use warm water or oil to immobilize the insect (see above). This may also flush the insect out of the ear. Even if the insect has been flushed out, you should have the ear examined by a doctor as soon as possible.

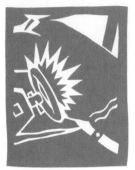

CHEST AND ABDOMINAL INJURIES

S EVERE CHEST AND ABDOMINAL injuries can be life-threatening. Immediate first-aid treatment is critical, especially if the injury is a wound that has penetrated the chest wall. Many people experience chest and abdominal injuries in automobile accidents. Knives, bullets, and other forms of blunt or penetrating force can also cause serious internal and external injuries to the chest and abdomen. Prompt medical care for the victim is essential.

Pneumothorax and hemothorax
In some sucking chest wounds (in which air flows in and out of the wound), air can become trapped between the chest wall and the lung (a condition known as pneumothorax) and may cause the lung to collapse. Hemothorax, a condition in which blood collects between the lungs and the chest wall, can also cause the lungs to collapse.

Injuries that crush the chest and abdomen are common in automobile accidents. These types of injuries are usually caused by compression of the driver's body against the steering wheel. Wearing seat belts dramatically reduces the incidence and severity of crushing injuries in automobile accidents. Crushing injuries are also common among pedestrians who are hit or run over by a vehicle.

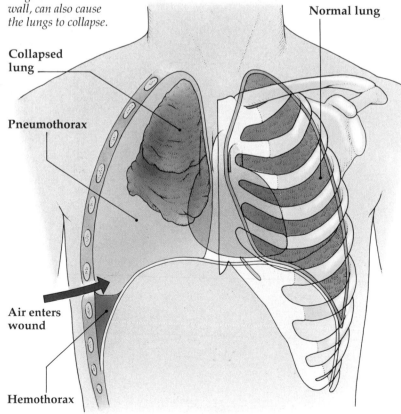

Normal lung

Collapsed lung

Pneumothorax

Air enters wound

Hemothorax

CHEST INJURIES

Fractures of the ribs and sternum (breastbone) may cause flail chest, pneumothorax and hemothorax (see left), and internal bleeding. Flail chest is a potentially fatal condition that may occur when several ribs are fractured. In flail chest, the damaged part of the rib cage is sucked inward when the person breathes in. This prevents the lungs from expanding and interferes with the movement of air into the lungs.

Penetrating chest wounds
Penetrating chest wounds can cause rib fractures; ends of fractured ribs may penetrate the pleura (the membrane that lines the chest cavity and covers the lungs) or lungs. In a person with a penetrating chest wound that punctures the lungs, breathing may result in air flowing in and out of the wound rather than the lungs. This condition is called a sucking chest wound (see left). In some penetrating chest wounds, the heart may be damaged, leading to bleeding into the pericardium (the fibrous bag that covers the heart). Bleeding into the pericardium can compress the heart, which prevents the heart from pumping blood. A cut into the heart or the main artery out of the heart can cause almost immediate death from severe internal bleeding.

FIRST AID FOR CHEST WOUNDS

A deep, open chest wound is a serious emergency. This type of injury may interfere with normal breathing and result in inadequate transfer of oxygen from the lungs, leading to an insufficient supply of oxygen to the brain. Signs and symptoms of chest injuries include rapid, noisy, and difficult breathing; blueness of the lips; collapse of the chest when the person breathes in; bruises on the chest; a crackling sensation when the chest is touched; and independent movement of part of the chest wall.

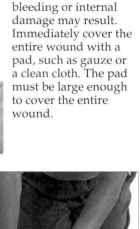

1 Have someone call an ambulance immediately. Do not remove any object that is embedded in the wound because serious bleeding or internal damage may result. Immediately cover the entire wound with a pad, such as gauze or a clean cloth. The pad must be large enough to cover the entire wound.

2 If no pad is available, place a hand on each side of the wound and firmly push the skin together to close the wound.

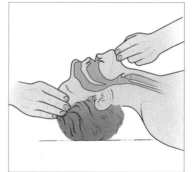

3 Apply a bandage with adhesive tape or other suitable material. If the person has difficulty breathing, untape one side of the bandage and pull the bandage away from the wound so that air trapped in the chest cavity can be expelled. If this precaution is not taken, a life-threatening pneumothorax (see page 80) may develop.

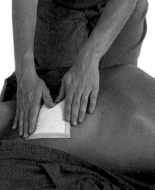

4 Maintain an open airway and restore breathing by artificial ventilation if necessary (see page 47). Keep the person comfortably warm to prevent shock (see page 57).

5 You may need to raise the person's shoulder slightly to help him or her breathe.

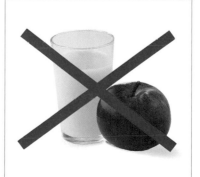

6 Do not give the person anything to eat or drink because he or she may choke. Also, the person's stomach should be empty in case surgery is required.

ABDOMINAL INJURIES

Injuries to the abdomen can cause damage to the abdominal organs, the pelvic bones, the abdominal or pelvic muscles, or the blood vessels. Blunt injuries of the abdomen are more common than penetrating injuries. Blunt injuries are caused by a strong force against the abdomen, as may occur when a driver is propelled into the steering wheel in an automobile accident. If only the abdominal muscles are injured, the damage is rarely serious and usually heals well without treatment. The severity of possible internal damage depends on the strength of force applied. If the intestines are distended or the bladder is full, these organs may be ruptured by a minor impact.

Penetrating wounds

Wounds that penetrate the wall of the abdomen may be caused by sharp objects, such as knives, or by bullets. Penetrating wounds of the abdomen can cause much more extensive damage to the internal organs than the size of the wound may suggest. Because the intestines are coiled in the abdomen, a penetrating wound may pass through several loops of intestine. Infection is common and is caused by the penetrating object and by the nonsterile contents of the intestine entering the abdominal cavity, leading to peritonitis (inflammation of the membrane that lines the abdominal cavity and covers the abdominal organs). When solid organs, such as the liver and spleen, are ruptured or lacerated, internal bleeding is severe and can be fatal.

TYPES OF ABDOMINAL INJURIES

Any forceful blow to the abdomen can cause severe damage to internal organs.

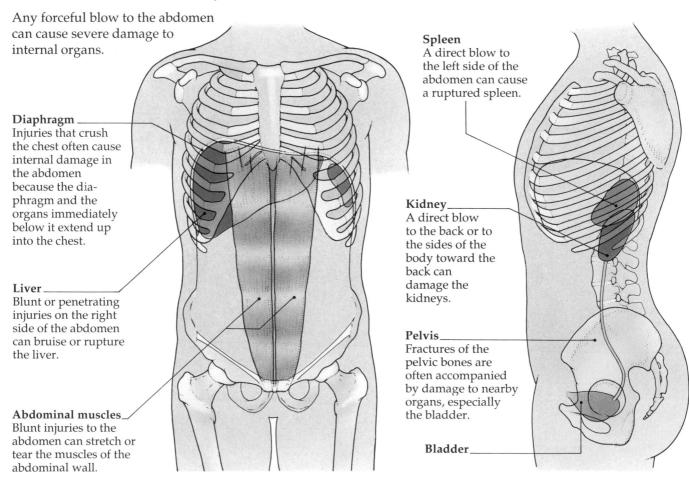

Diaphragm
Injuries that crush the chest often cause internal damage in the abdomen because the diaphragm and the organs immediately below it extend up into the chest.

Liver
Blunt or penetrating injuries on the right side of the abdomen can bruise or rupture the liver.

Abdominal muscles
Blunt injuries to the abdomen can stretch or tear the muscles of the abdominal wall.

Spleen
A direct blow to the left side of the abdomen can cause a ruptured spleen.

Kidney
A direct blow to the back or to the sides of the body toward the back can damage the kidneys.

Pelvis
Fractures of the pelvic bones are often accompanied by damage to nearby organs, especially the bladder.

Bladder

FIRST AID FOR ABDOMINAL INJURIES

Bleeding from an abdominal wound is often severe, and it is important to control the bleeding quickly. Severe internal bleeding from a damaged organ can very quickly become life-threatening.

1 Have someone call an ambulance immediately. Maintain an open airway and restore breathing by artificial ventilation if necessary (see page 47). Lay the person on his or her back. Bend the person's legs and place a pillow or rolled blanket or towel under the knees to relax the abdominal muscles.

2 Apply direct pressure if necessary to control bleeding. Do not try to remove embedded objects. If the intestines are protruding from the wound, do not try to push them back into the wound; cover them with a pad that has been soaked in clean water. Cover the entire wound with a sterile dressing or clean cloth.

3 Keep the person comfortably warm to prevent shock (see page 57). Do not give the person anything to eat or drink; his or her stomach should be empty because surgery will probably be necessary.

Signs of abdominal injury

One of the most common signs of abdominal injury is bruising. In some cases, the bruise reflects the pattern of the object that caused it, such as a steering wheel. This type of bruise may indicate a compression injury and is often accompanied by internal damage. However, the lack of such bruising in no way rules out serious internal injury.

The most common signs of internal injury are tenderness in the abdominal area and tightening of the abdominal muscles when gentle pressure is applied around the site of the injury. Pain caused by an abdominal injury tends to worsen with time. Sometimes, the abdomen becomes distended as a result of severe internal bleeding. Abdominal injuries that cause internal bleeding may also cause symptoms such as restlessness, apprehensiveness, thirst, confusion, abnormal paleness, and a rapid, weak pulse. The person may vomit blood. A ruptured liver or spleen may cause pain felt in the tip of the shoulder.

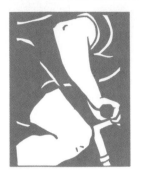

ARM AND LEG INJURIES

Y OUR ARMS AND LEGS are considerably more vulnerable to injury than other parts of your body. For example, almost half of all work-related injuries involve the arms, legs, hands, or feet. A strong force or excessive stress on your arms and legs can overload the bones or soft tissues and cause damage, such as a broken bone or a torn muscle or tendon.

SEVERE INJURIES

If a wound gapes, if you feel a "pins-and-needles" sensation, if you cannot move your fingers or toes, or if you notice signs of infection (such as redness, swelling, pus, or extreme tenderness around a wound), call your doctor immediately.

Minor scrapes and cuts often require only cleaning and bandaging. More serious injuries such as a deep cut or a broken bone require medical attention. The severity of the injury may not always be obvious. Someone's hand crushed in a piece of machinery, for example, may show little damage to the underlying bones, but the muscles, tendons, and blood vessels may be severely damaged. If you have any doubt about the extent of damage caused by an injury, see your doctor as soon as possible.

BASEBALL FINGER

Baseball finger occurs when a blow to the end of a finger or a severe bending strain tears the tendon from the bone or the bone breaks at the point where the tendon is attached. Apply a cold pack to prevent swelling and stop internal bleeding. Your doctor will apply a splint. In some cases, surgery is needed.

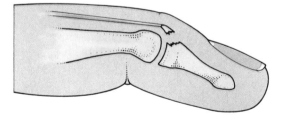

Torn tendon
The tendon is torn from the bone, breaking off a small fragment of bone.

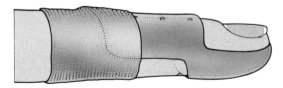

Splint
The splint immobilizes the injured finger.

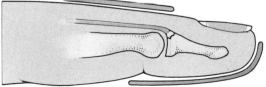

Healed tendon
It usually takes about 4 to 8 weeks for the torn tendon to heal.

CRUSH INJURIES

Crush injuries may be caused by smashing your fingers in a closing car door or cabinet door. Crush injuries also occur if furniture or heavy objects are dropped on toes or a finger is hit with a heavy object such as a hammer. X-rays may be necessary with crush injuries to check for broken bones. Immediate first aid for a crush injury includes applying cold packs to help relieve pain and swelling, and immobilizing (usually with a splint) the injured part of the body. Elevate the injured limb above the level of the heart to help control swelling, and call your doctor as soon as possible.

WOUNDS

All deep wounds (see WARNING on page 88) of the hand, wrist, arm, leg, and foot should be checked by your doctor as soon as possible so that he or she can evaluate the extent of internal damage caused by the injury. Surgery may be required to repair internal damage.

Hand and wrist

Deep wounds on the hand or wrist may damage the nerves, blood vessels, and tendons beneath the surface of the skin. When a tendon is cut, there may be partial or even complete loss of function. For example, if you have a deep wound on the back of your hand and you cannot straighten your fingers, one or more tendons may have been cut.

Nerve injury in the wrist
Even a small puncture wound in the wrist – such as may be caused by a piece of broken glass – can cut the median nerve, which controls some of the muscles in the hand.

Blood vessel

Wrist bones

Tendons

Median nerve

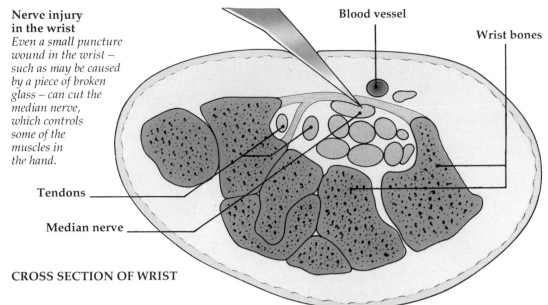

CROSS SECTION OF WRIST

Knee

Deep wounds to the knee should be examined by your doctor as soon as possible. If the wound penetrates to the joint and the joint becomes infected, arthritis may develop as a result of the infection in the joint. Deep wounds on the side of the knee may damage the ligaments (tough tissue that binds bone ends together) and cause the knee joint to become unstable. If you have a deep wound below the kneecap, the tendon may be severed and you may be unable to straighten the injured leg.

NAIL INJURIES

Hitting your fingertip with a hammer or slamming it in a door may break small blood vessels under the nail, causing a blood clot to form. Within 1 or 2 days, the fingernail turns black and the pressure of the blood clot may cause extreme pain.

Blood clot under a fingernail
Your doctor will gently puncture the blood clot to allow blood to drain by inserting a needle through the fingernail or under the fingernail into the clot.

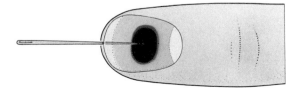

See your doctor if the nail is severely damaged or if a blood clot forms (see below). Never disturb a damaged nail other than to trim it. If the fingernail becomes loose, protect it with a bandage; do not pull it off. As the new fingernail grows, it will push off the damaged fingernail. Similar injuries to toenails should be treated in the same way.

SPLINTERS

Remove splinters with a sterilized needle and tweezers. If the splinter is protruding, pull it out with the tweezers at the same angle as the splinter entered the skin. If the splinter is visible below the skin, loosen the skin around the splinter with the needle until you can grasp the splinter with the tweezers and remove it. Squeeze the wound so it bleeds to help remove bacteria and debris. Wash the wound with soap and water for at least 5 minutes and put a bandage on the wound. Check the wound during the next few days for redness, pus, and red streaks leading from the wound, which indicate infection. If the splinter breaks off in the wound or is deeply embedded, see your doctor as soon as possible for removal of the splinter and possibly a tetanus booster shot.

FISHHOOKS
Never attempt to remove a fishhook caught in the eye or face; get medical help immediately. The illustrations below show how to remove a fishhook embedded in a finger. After removing the fishhook, clean the entry and exit wounds with soap and water and then bandage the wounds. See your doctor as soon as possible; you may need a tetanus booster shot.

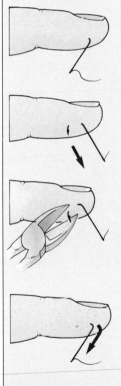

Removing a fishhook
Push the fishhook through the skin until the barb comes out. Cut the hook with pliers or clippers either at the barb or at the shank. Carefully remove the remaining part of the fishhook.

BANDAGING AND SPLINTING

If you suspect that a person has a broken arm or leg, first control any external bleeding and then immobilize the injured limb with a splint before moving the person. If a person with a broken bone is moved without immobilizing the injury, the ends of the broken bones may damage nerves or blood vessels.

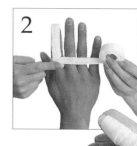

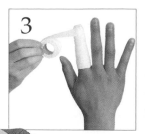

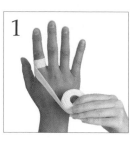

BANDAGING

Buddy strapping

"Buddy strapping" is a technique used to immobilize injured fingers and toes. Place a gauze pad between the injured finger or toe and the adjacent digit; then tape the two digits together.

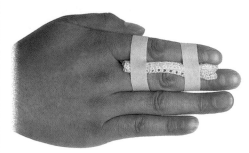

Fingertip bandaging

Fasten the bandage loosely at the base of the finger with several circular turns (1). Bring the bandage up the front of the finger, over the fingertip, and down the back to the base of the finger. Hold the bandage at the base and repeat the back-and-forth bandaging over the fingertip several times (2). Starting at the base of the finger, wrap the bandage around the finger, working up to the fingertip and back down to the base (3). Apply adhesive tape that runs up the finger, over the fingertip, and down the other side (4).

Figure-of-eight bandaging

Fasten the bandage with one or two circular turns (1). Wrap the bandage diagonally across the foot, around the heel and ankle (2). Continue the bandage across the top of the foot and under the arch (3). Repeat the figure-of-eight turns, with each turn overlapping the previous turn by about three quarters of the width of the bandage, wrapping the bandage until the foot and ankle are covered (4).

Circular bandaging

Circular bandaging is often used on wrist, toe, and finger injuries. Fasten the bandage by placing one end of the gauze at an angle over the dressing (1), making several circular turns to hold the dressing and the end of the bandage in place (2). Continue to wrap the bandage and overlap each turn until the dressing is covered, then secure the bandage with adhesive tape or tie a knot in the gauze (3).

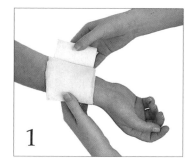

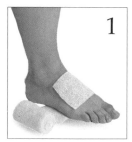

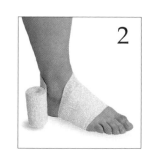

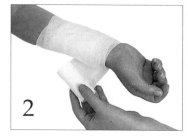

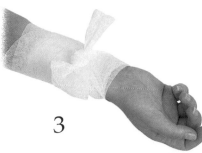

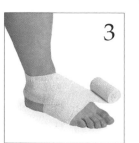

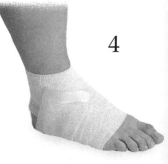

SPLINTING

Upper arm
Place light padding under the person's armpit. Then place the arm at the person's side, with the lower part of the arm at a right angle across the chest. Put a padded splint on the outside of the arm and tie it in place above and below the injured area, with the knots on the outside; support the lower part of the arm on a narrow sling tied around the neck (1). Wrap a sheet or large towel around the person's chest and back and tie it under the opposite arm (2). (See page 68 for lower-arm and wrist injuries.)

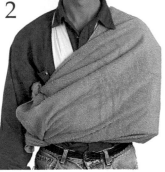

Elbow
Do not try to straighten an injured elbow. If the elbow is bent, follow the procedures at left for the two slings applied for upper-arm injuries. If the elbow is straight, do not bend it. Put padding in the person's armpit and apply padded splints on both sides of the arm (see right). If splints are not available, immobilize the injured elbow as shown below.

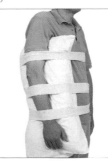

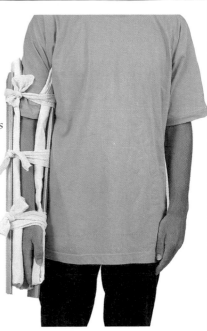

Hand
Place a padded splint underneath the lower part of the arm and hand and tie the splint in place. Gently place the lower part of the arm and elbow at a right angle to the person's chest (1). Elevate the hand about 4 inches above the elbow. Put the lower part of the arm in a sling and tie the sling around the neck (2).

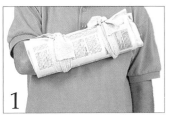

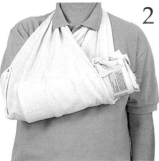

Ankle and foot
Put a pillow (or a towel or rolled blanket) around the leg from the calf to beyond the heel (1). Tie the pillow in place and fold the end beyond the heel up to support the foot (2).

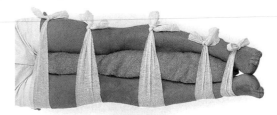

Upper leg (thigh)
Carefully straighten the knee of the injured leg. Place padding between the person's legs. If you do not have splints, tie the injured leg to the uninjured leg in several places, but not over the injured area (see below). If you have splints, slip seven long bandages under the person's body at the ankles; above and below the knees;

Kneecap
Gently straighten the injured leg, if possible. Place a padded board at least 4 inches wide under the leg. The board should reach from the heel to beyond the buttocks. Tie the splint in place at the ankle, just above and below the knee, and at the thigh.

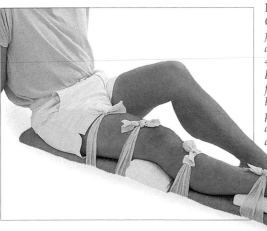

at the thigh, pelvis, and lower back; and just below the armpits. Place one splint on the outside of the injured leg, reaching from the armpit to below the heel. Place the other splint on the inside of the injured leg, reaching from the crotch to below the heel. Tie the splints to the injured leg. (See page 68 for splinting lower-leg injuries.)

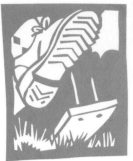

WOUNDS, CUTS, AND ABRASIONS

OPEN WOUNDS ARE THE RESULT of injuries that tear the skin. Most wounds are not serious and can be cleaned with soap and water and then covered with a sterile dressing or adhesive bandage. Severe wounds often require medical attention to control bleeding and to prevent infection and severe scarring.

Everyone gets a minor cut or abrasion from time to time. First-aid treatment for these types of minor injuries is important to ensure that the wound will not become infected and will heal quickly.

TYPES OF WOUNDS

An open wound is an injury in which the skin is broken and bleeding. A break in the skin surface can lead to infection if the wound is not cleaned properly. Keep all wounds clean and watch for signs of possible infection, such as fever, redness, heat or swelling at the wound, pus beneath the skin or in the wound, or red streaks leading from the wound. Signs of infection usually occur 24 to 72 hours after the injury. If a wound becomes infected, see your doctor immediately.

Puncture wounds

A puncture wound results from penetration of the skin by a sharp object. There is usually little bleeding, which increases the chance of infection because bacteria and debris are not washed out.

Cuts

A cut may be a clean, straight incision in the skin caused by a sharp object, such as a knife or a piece of glass, or may be a rough, jagged tear in the skin (called a laceration) caused by an object with sharp, irregular edges, such as a rock.

Abrasions

Abrasions are damage to the skin as a result of a scrape against a hard surface, usually resulting in little bleeding from the wound but possible infection.

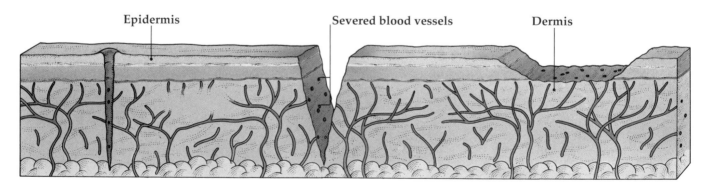

Epidermis   Severed blood vessels   Dermis

Treating puncture wounds
Always consult your doctor if you have a puncture wound. Puncture wounds may damage tendons, nerves, and blood vessels. Do not remove deeply embedded objects; this may cause more damage. Flush the wound with running water to help remove debris.

Treating cuts
If a cut is bleeding severely, apply direct pressure (see page 89). A butterfly bandage or stitches may be used to keep the edges of the cut together (see page 133). A severe cut may damage tendons, nerves, and blood vessels and requires medical treatment.

Treating abrasions
Thoroughly clean and remove all dirt and other foreign material (such as small stones or grit) from an abrasion (see page 89). Any foreign material remaining in an abrasion can cause infection.

HOW TO TREAT MINOR WOUNDS, CUTS, AND ABRASIONS

1 Always wash your hands with soap and water before you treat a wound.

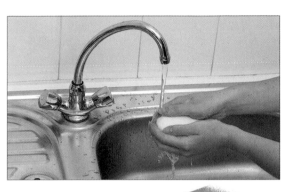

2 If a cut is bleeding, apply direct pressure over the wound with a sterile pad or clean cloth until bleeding has stopped.

3 Wash the wound with soap and water. Rinse the wound under running water. You may need to gently scrub the area to remove any dirt, or use sterilized tweezers to remove foreign material near the skin's surface. Do not try to remove any deeply embedded particles.

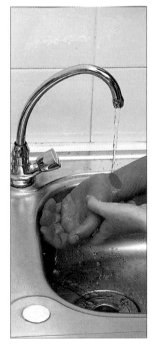

4 Pat the wound dry with a sterile pad or clean cloth. Do not use cotton balls or a cloth with fibers that may stick to the wound.

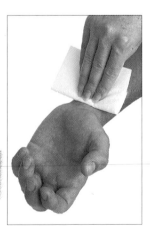

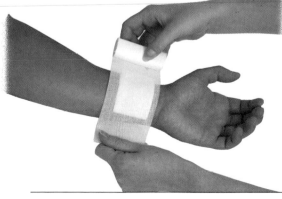

5 Cover the wound with a sterile dressing or bandage.

WOUNDS, CUTS, AND ABRASIONS

Q I fell while I was working in my garden, and a sharp twig that was buried in the soil went through my gardening glove and got stuck in my hand. The spot hardly bled after I pulled out the twig, but my doctor still gave me a booster tetanus shot. Why?

A A booster tetanus shot was essential if you had not been immunized within the last 5 to 10 years. Spores of tetanus bacteria live in the soil. Your wound was potentially dangerous because contaminated particles may have been forced deep into the wound by the twig.

Q My son cut himself and had to have stitches. Because the stitches hurt him, he is afraid to go back to the doctor to have them removed. What should I do?

A Removing stitches may cause some discomfort, but you can reassure your son that getting the stitches removed should not hurt as much as having them put in. Your son may feel a slight pinching sensation if the stitches have stuck to the scab or newly formed skin.

Q What can I do to control bleeding from a wound if I don't have any sterile pads or bandages? Also, is it necessary to sterilize tweezers before using them?

A If sterile pads are not available, any clean cloth or clothing item can be used if direct pressure is needed to control bleeding. Tweezers kept in a medicine cabinet are not usually contaminated. If you want to sterilize the tweezers, boil them in water for 10 minutes.

BURNS AND ELECTRICAL INJURIES

EVERY YEAR ABOUT 2 million people are burned or scalded severely enough to need medical treatment. Most burns are the result of accidents in the home. Burn injuries most commonly occur among children and older people. An electrical injury can cause severe burns and life-threatening damage to internal organs.

Burns may be caused by flame, hot objects, chemicals, electric currents, or radiation. Scalds are injuries caused by hot liquids and high-temperature gases such as steam. About 75 percent of deaths from burns are caused by house fires, more than half of which are started by careless cigarette smoking. Most burns that are caused by accidental contact with chemicals occur in the workplace. The most common burn injury caused by radiation is sunburn.

TYPES OF BURNS

If the skin is exposed to a temperature above 120°F (49°C) for even a short time, skin cells are damaged. Burns and scalds are categorized by the severity of damage to the skin.

CHEMICAL BURNS TO THE SKIN

Contact with some chemicals can cause severe damage to tissues, particularly the eyes (see page 77). For chemical burns to the skin, flush the affected area with slowly running cold water for at least 5 minutes. Continue to flush with water while removing clothing from the burned area. Cover the burn with a sterile bandage or a nonfluffy clean cloth; cool, wet dressings are best to soothe pain. Seek immediate medical help.

First-degree burns
First-degree burns affect only the outer layer of the skin (the epidermis). These burns cause redness, blistering, and peeling of the surface layers of skin cells that have been killed. Sunburn and brief contact with hot objects are common causes of first-degree burns.

Second-degree burns
Second-degree burns cause injury into the layer of skin beneath the epidermis (the dermis). These burns cause severe pain and swelling but permanent scarring does not usually occur. Severe sunburn, hot liquids, and flash burns from gasoline are common causes of second-degree burns.

Third-degree burns
Third-degree burns destroy the epidermis and the dermis. The skin looks white or charred. If the burn is deep, the fatty layer beneath the skin (including muscles and bones) may be affected. Fire, prolonged contact with hot objects or liquids, and electrical burns are common causes of third-degree burns.

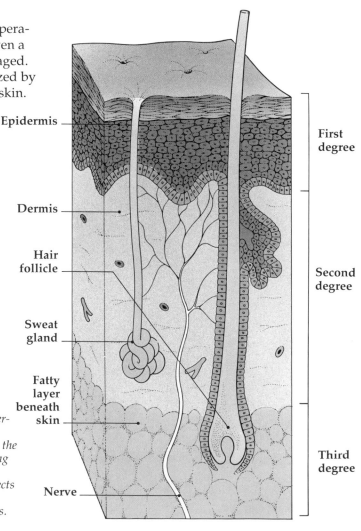

Epidermis

Dermis

Hair follicle

Sweat gland

Fatty layer beneath skin

Nerve

First degree

Second degree

Third degree

FIRST AID FOR BURNS

Treatment of burns and scalds depends on the severity of the injury. The initial first-aid treatment of burns reduces the temperature of the burned area, which helps prevent further injury to the skin and underlying tissues. Never apply ointments, sprays, antiseptics, or home remedies such as butter to a burn. For first-aid treatment of electrical burns, see page 93.

FIRST-DEGREE BURNS

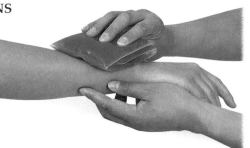

1 Immediately place the burned area under cold running water or apply a cold-water compress until pain subsides.

2 Cover the burn with a sterile bandage or nonfluffy clean cloth.

SECOND-DEGREE BURNS

1 Second-degree burns need immediate medical treatment. Put the burned area in cold water or apply towels or rags that have been soaked in cold water. Cover the burned area with a sterile nonfluffy bandage or clean cloth. Do not attempt to break any blisters.

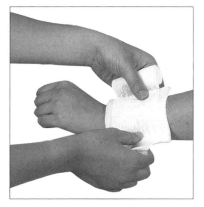

2 If the burn is to the mouth and throat, take the person to the emergency department immediately. Breathing may become difficult because the throat may swell quickly, possibly closing the airway. Give the person sips of cold water at frequent intervals and remove any constricting clothing or jewelry.

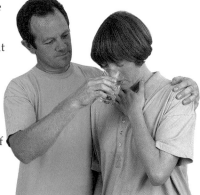

THIRD-DEGREE BURNS

1 Third-degree burns (even small ones) require immediate medical treatment. If the person is on fire, smother the flames with a blanket or jacket. Be sure to smother the flames from the neck downward; otherwise you may force the flames toward the person's face.

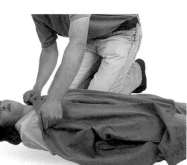

2 Make certain that the person is breathing. Breathing difficulties often follow smoke inhalation and burns around the face, neck, and mouth.

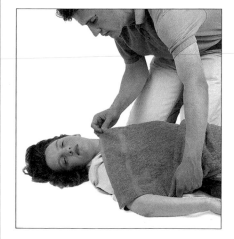

3 Place a cold cloth or gently pour cool or cold water on the burned area. Do not place ice on the burn. Cover the burned area with a thick, sterile, nonfluffy dressing. Do not remove anything that is stuck to a burn.

4 Elevate burned arms or legs and keep the person lying down. If the person has face or neck burns, prop the person's back and shoulders up with pillows; check often to see if the person has trouble breathing.

ELECTRICAL INJURIES

About 4,000 electricity-related injuries occur each year, causing about 1,000 deaths. About one third of all electrical injuries occur in the home; the remainder occur among workers in electricity-generating or construction industries. The passage of an electric current through the body can disrupt the electrical activity in the brain that controls breathing. A severe electric shock can cause the heart to fibrillate (quiver in a rapid, irregular pattern) or stop beating.

Tissue damage

The amount of damage to body tissues caused by an electric shock depends on the electrical voltage that is applied to the body and the body's resistance to current flow. The higher the voltage and the stronger the flow of electrical current that passes through the body, the more extensive the burns may be. Your skin has a high resistance to current flow. Water is an excellent conductor of electricity, so, if your skin is wet, your resistance to the flow of the electrical current is substantially lowered and the risk of electrical injury is much greater.

PREVENTING ELECTRICAL INJURY

You can reduce the risk of electrical injury by taking the following safety precautions:

Electrical appliances
Many electrical injuries result from defects in electrical appliances. Never attempt to make electrical repairs on home appliances yourself – this type of work should always be done by a qualified electrician.

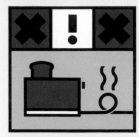

Electrical outlets
Young children are particularly at risk from injuries caused by electrical outlets. To prevent your child from poking objects into the socket, put covers on all electrical outlets when they are not in use. Do not use any metal tool or implement on an electrical appliance that is plugged in; always unplug the appliance first.

Electricity and water
Water is an excellent conductor of electricity. Do not use an electrical appliance, such as a hair dryer, near a sink or bathtub. Never place vases or other objects that contain water on an electrical appliance, such as a television. Be particularly careful of wet surfaces and spilled liquids when using electrical appliances in the kitchen.

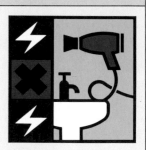

Recommended safe distance from victim is 60 feet

High-voltage electricity
Contact with high-voltage electricity in power lines is usually immediately fatal. Never attempt to rescue a victim of an electrical injury from a high-voltage power source until the power has been turned off – the electricity may arc and jump a considerable distance. Call for medical help immediately.

Signs and symptoms

The victim of an electrical injury may have severe burns visible where the electric current entered the body, as well as where the current left the body. There may be extensive internal damage between these points; severe internal injuries may exist with only minimal external signs of damage. A severe electrical injury may disrupt the breathing and circulatory centers in the brain; breathing may become difficult, or breathing and heartbeat may stop simultaneously. The person may show signs of shock (see page 57). If the injury is caused by lightning, bones may have broken as a result of sudden, strong muscle contractions or being thrown into the air and onto the ground by the force of the lightning.

FIRST AID FOR ELECTRICAL INJURIES

A severe electric shock can knock a person to the ground. He or she may lose consciousness and may stop breathing, and his or her heart may stop beating. A person who has received a severe electrical shock should always be examined by a doctor; internal damage can occur that may not be immediately apparent. If you witness an electrical accident or you are the first at the scene, your first step is to separate the person from the source of electricity. First aid for victims of an electrical shock is given below.

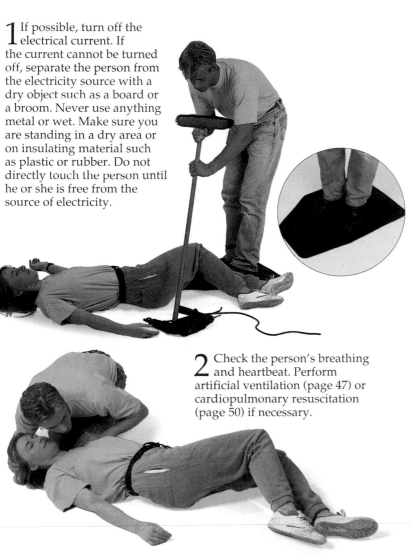

1 If possible, turn off the electrical current. If the current cannot be turned off, separate the person from the electricity source with a dry object such as a board or a broom. Never use anything metal or wet. Make sure you are standing in a dry area or on insulating material such as plastic or rubber. Do not directly touch the person until he or she is free from the source of electricity.

2 Check the person's breathing and heartbeat. Perform artificial ventilation (page 47) or cardiopulmonary resuscitation (page 50) if necessary.

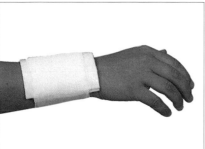

3 Once the person is breathing, call for medical help immediately. Cover burns with dry, loose dressings and then a bandage. Do not break blisters or remove any loose skin, and do not apply any lotions or ointments to the burn. If necessary, treat for bleeding and shock (see page 54) and for any broken bones (see page 66).

AVOIDING LIGHTNING STRIKES

Lightning causes about 1,000 injuries and between 250 and 300 deaths each year. You can reduce your risk of being struck by lightning by quickly getting inside a building during a thunderstorm. If you cannot get indoors, move to the lowest ground possible. Remember the following safety tips:

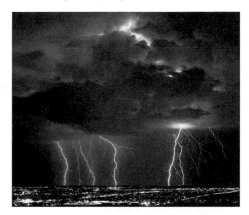

◆ Do not seek shelter under a high structure such as a tree – high structures attract lightning. Avoid open ground where you are the tallest object.

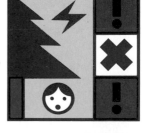

◆ If you are playing golf or fishing, drop your clubs or fishing pole immediately – they can act as lightning conductors.

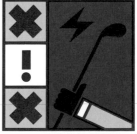

◆ Do not open your umbrella – it can act as a lightning rod.

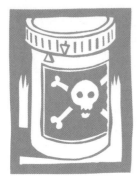

POISONING

Poisons are substances – solids, liquids, and gases – that can cause temporary or permanent damage in the body by disrupting the function and structure of cells. Poisons can be swallowed, inhaled, or absorbed through the skin. Some poisons act quickly; others are slow-acting and may not cause signs or symptoms right away. Always call your local poison control center immediately for first-aid instructions when treating a poisoning victim.

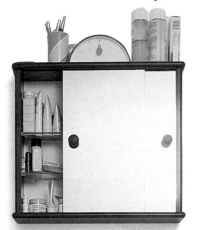

Approximately 1 million poisonings are reported each year. Children have a compelling urge to explore, and they can reach the most surprising places. More than 75 percent of all poisonings occur in children under the age of 5. In children, the poisonous substances are usually household cleaning products. In adults, poisoning is often the result of an accidental drug overdose or a very high dose of vitamin and mineral supplements. In addition to poisons being swallowed, inhaled, or absorbed through the skin, poisons may also be injected under the skin by insects and snakes (see page 116).

MEDICATIONS AND HOUSEHOLD PRODUCTS

Keep all medications out of the reach of children – even those medications that are made especially for children. Overdoses of prescription or over-the-counter drugs can be extremely dangerous. Excessive doses of familiar and seemingly harmless medications such as aspirin and acetaminophen can cause serious or even life-threatening adverse effects in both children and adults.

To minimize your risk of a drug-related poisoning, never take more than the recommended dose unless your doctor tells you to, and never take your medications in the dark – you might take the wrong medication or the wrong dose.

Avoiding poisonous gases
Inhaling carbon monoxide causes more poisoning deaths than any other inhaled substance. Carbon monoxide is usually inhaled as a result of poor ventilation, faulty kerosene space heaters, and malfunctioning furnaces. Keep all rooms in your house well ventilated, never leave the engine of a car or motorcycle running in a closed garage, and have your furnace cleaned and checked once a year.

Preventing drug poisoning
Keep all drugs and medications out of the reach of children. Medications used to relieve teething pain are made to have a pleasant, sweet taste. Some of these medications contain benzocaine, a drug that can cause a life-threatening reaction if your child eats even small quantities.

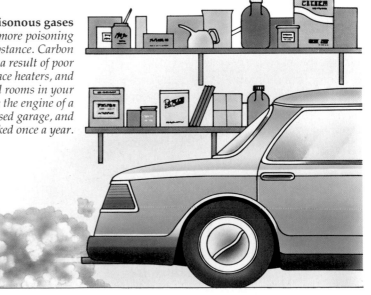

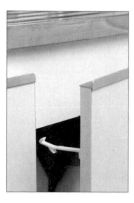

Safe storage
Store household cleaning and gardening products in a locked or childproof cabinet or out of reach of children. Never store these products in the same places as food or drink. Even adults can accidentally poison themselves with products that are stored in improperly labeled containers.

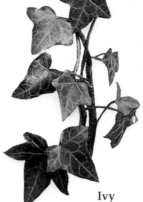

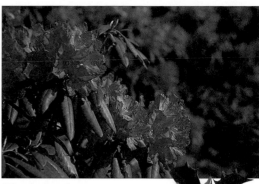

Ivy   Rhododendron

Also, never take medications that were prescribed for someone else, even if you think you have the same illness.

Household and gardening products, such as bleach, detergents, drain openers, weed killers, and insecticides, are common causes of poisoning emergencies. Always keep these products in a childproof or locked cabinet (see above). When you are using these chemicals, never leave them unattended when children are around. Some substances, such as insecticides, can cause serious harm if they come into contact with the skin. If swallowed, toiletries such as shaving cream, nail polish, and perfume can cause unpleasant and sometimes severe adverse reactions.

ALCOHOL

Alcohol, which is a drug, is potentially poisonous. Always keep alcohol in a locked cabinet or in a place that children cannot reach. The ethanol in alcoholic beverages slows down the activity of the central nervous system (the brain and spinal cord). Alcohol consumption can cause lack of coordination and slowed reactions, slurred speech, abnormal breathing, lethargy (tiredness, drowsiness, or lack of energy), or possible coma. Drinking large quantities of alcohol can damage your body in many ways, both temporarily and permanently. For example, liver damage is a serious and common consequence of the long-term poisonous effects of drinking alcoholic beverages.

PLANTS AND MUSHROOMS

Many plants and mushrooms are poisonous. Teach your children not to eat any mushrooms or plants they find outdoors. Children are frequently poisoned as a result of eating colorful berries from plants. If you pick wild mushrooms, be sure they are not poisonous. Most fatal cases of mushroom poisoning are caused by the *Amanita phalloides* mushroom, which looks similar to an edible mushroom.

Holly

Poisonous plants and mushrooms
Many poisonous plants are brightly colored and can attract the attention of children. Common poisonous plants are rhododendron, ivy, and holly (above). Poisoning by the colorful mushroom Amanita muscaria *(left) produces symptoms very rapidly. Although poisoning by this mushroom is rarely severe in adults, ingestion of large quantities of the mushroom by young children may cause seizures and coma.*

SYMPTOMS OF POISONING

Different types of poisons affect the body in different ways and produce a wide variety of symptoms. If you witness a poisoning or suspect that someone has been poisoned, call your local poison control center immediately for first-aid instructions (see below), even if the person does not seem to have any symptoms. Some poisons take time to have an effect; symptoms may not appear until some time after poisoning.

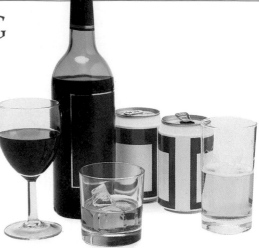

Carbon monoxide
Symptoms and signs of carbon monoxide poisoning may include headache, nausea, vomiting, dilated pupils, and abnormally flushed or "cherry red" skin. The person may become confused, lose consciousness, and die.

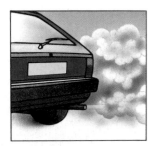

Alcohol
The short-term effects of excess alcohol include nausea and vomiting, headache, blackouts, and unconsciousness. The most common long-term effect of persistent heavy alcohol consumption is liver damage; other parts of the body, such as the heart and brain, can also be affected.

Mushrooms
Poisoning by the Amanita phalloides *mushroom causes severe abdominal pain, vomiting, and diarrhea. Ten to 15 percent of people poisoned by this mushroom die of liver failure. Other symptoms of mushroom poisoning are drowsiness, vision problems, muscle tremors (trembling or shaking), and delirium (mental confusion). Symptoms usually occur 6 hours or more after eating a poisonous mushroom.*

Drugs other than alcohol
A drug overdose may cause drowsiness, unconsciousness, shallow or irregular breathing, vomiting, or seizures. Symptoms can occur within a short time or may develop hours or days later.

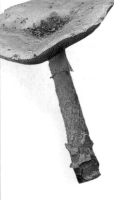

Poisonous plants
Symptoms of poisoning by plants vary but may include abdominal pain, vomiting, flushing, breathing difficulties, delirium (mental confusion), and unconsciousness.

FIRST AID FOR POISONING

Always call your local poison control center immediately for first-aid instructions. Be sure to give the person's age, the name of the poison, how much poison was swallowed and how long ago, whether the person has vomited, and how long it will take to get to the nearest hospital emergency department.

1 Do not give the person any fluids to try to dilute the poison unless you are instructed to do so. Induce vomiting (with syrup of ipecac) only if you are told to do this. Keep the person sitting up or lying face down to prevent choking if vomiting occurs.

2 If the person has been poisoned by absorption through the skin (for example, by an insecticide), wash the skin thoroughly with soap and water to remove as much of the poison as possible. Always wear gloves when removing contaminated clothing.

Methyl alcohol

Methyl alcohol (also called wood alcohol or methanol) is found in paint, paint thinner, varnish, and antifreeze. If a person drinks it, a severe chemical imbalance, blindness, and collapse of the circulatory system can result. The person's breath may have an alcoholic odor.

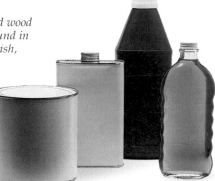

Fluorocarbons and toluene

Some people intentionally inhale fluorocarbons (used in some aerosol sprays) and toluene (used in glues) to get high. Symptoms of poisoning by these substances may include hallucinations, panic, lethargy (tiredness, drowsiness, or lack of energy), and coma.

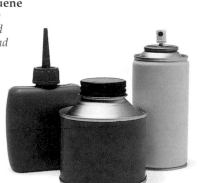

Absorbed poisons

Some poisons can be absorbed through the skin. For example, absorption of organophosphates, which are in most insecticides, causes nausea, sweating, a feeling of tightness in the chest, abdominal cramps, and excessive salivation. In severe cases, seizures may occur and breathing may stop.

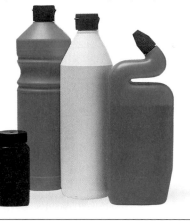

Chemicals

Swallowing chemicals, such as drain openers, toilet bowl cleaners, rust removers, detergents, and bleach, can cause burns in the mouth and throat, resulting in difficulty swallowing.

Petroleum products

Swallowing petroleum products, such as kerosene, gasoline, and lighter fluid, can cause severe breathing difficulties. Poisoning victims may also have severe abdominal pain or symptoms such as delirium (mental confusion) and lethargy (tiredness, drowsiness, or lack of energy).

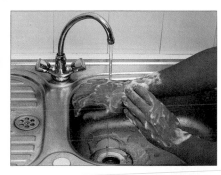

4 If the person is unconscious, do not give any fluids and do not try to induce vomiting. If the person is not breathing, open the person's airway and begin artificial ventilation if necessary (see page 47). Start cardiopulmonary resuscitation (see page 50) if the person's heart has stopped beating.

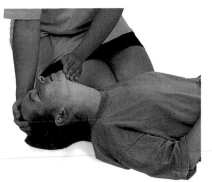

3 If the person has inhaled a poisonous gas, get him or her into fresh air immediately and loosen any tight clothing around the person's neck and waist.

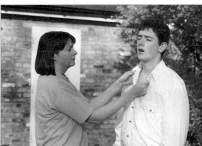

5 Give medical personnel any items found near the person – such as drugs or medications, empty containers or bottles, or plants – to help them determine the appropriate treatment.

CASE HISTORY
A CURIOUS CHILD

B**RAD AND HIS MOTHER were visiting his grandfather. While the adults were cleaning out the garage, Brad went inside to watch television. He got bored with the program and went into the kitchen to get something to drink. On the kitchen counter, Brad saw a drinking glass with bright orange pills in it that looked like orange candy.**

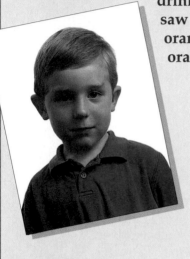

PERSONAL DETAILS
Name Brad Hutchinson
Age 5
Occupation Kindergarten student
Family Brad's parents are divorced.

THE INCIDENT
Brad eats several of the pills but puts the rest back on the kitchen counter because they don't taste good. He drinks a glass of juice and then goes back to watch television.

FIRST AID
Brad's mother, Elaine, comes into the house to check on Brad and sees that he has fallen asleep in front of the television. When she tries to wake him, he does not respond. Elaine checks to see that Brad is still breathing and runs into the kitchen to call an ambulance. She notices the pills on the kitchen counter near Brad's juice glass and she is afraid Brad must have mistaken the pills for candy. She yells to her father, Mike, for help. Mike immediately calls the poison control center and tells them that his grandson has swallowed several amitriptyline pills (an antidepressant). The poison control center tells Mike to keep Brad lying on his side in case he begins to vomit.

AT THE HOSPITAL
The doctor in the emergency department examines Brad, who is still unconscious. The doctor puts a tube down Brad's throat to keep his airway open while another tube is put into Brad's stomach to wash out the pills. Activated charcoal is given through the tube into his stomach to adsorb any of the medication that

may still be in his stomach. An intravenous line is inserted in his right arm for administration of fluids and medications if needed. The doctor monitors Brad's heart with an electrocardiogram. Brad's mother and grandfather then talk to the doctor about how the accident occurred. Mike explains that he took the pills out of their container because the arthritis in his fingers makes it hard for him to remove the childproof cap. The doctor reminds Mike that medications should always be kept in their original containers. The doctor recommends that Mike ask his pharmacist to put his medication in containers with easy-to-open caps designed for people with arthritis, and that Mike keep these bottles in a locked cabinet.

THE OUTCOME
Brad's condition is closely watched overnight. The next morning Brad is conscious but still drowsy and confused. He gets better in time and is able to go home in a few days.

Monitoring Brad's heart
In the emergency department, electrocardiograph leads are attached to Brad's chest. Brad's heartbeat is monitored because an overdose of amitriptyline can cause serious heart arrhythmias (irregular heartbeats).

**Giving oxygen
for poisoning**
*Some poisons (such as
carbon monoxide) affect
the amount of oxygen in
the bloodstream. Oxygen
may be given through a
mask to ensure an ad-
equate supply of oxygen
and to help remove the
carbon monoxide from
the person's system.*

SEIZURES

Some types of
poisons, particu-
larly some drugs,
can cause seizures.
Seizures are
uncontrolled
muscle contrac-
tions. If someone
has a seizure, call
for medical help
immediately. Do
not try to hold the
person down;
move furniture and
other hazards out
of the way so that
the person cannot
injure himself or
herself. Do not give
the person any-
thing to drink, and
do not try to
induce vomiting.
If the person
vomits, turn his or
her head to the
side so that he or
she will not choke
on the vomit.

MEDICAL TREATMENT OF POISONING

A doctor chooses the most effective
treatment of poisoning based on the type
of poison. An antidote (a substance that
neutralizes the poison) can be given for
some poisons. If you can identify the
poison and the amount taken, this information could save the person's life.

Pumping the stomach

The treatment of people who have swallowed poisons may include gastric
lavage, in which the contents of the
stomach are washed out (see page 132).
After washing the poison out of the
stomach, activated charcoal is usually
given. Charcoal adsorbs many substances, including drugs and poisons,
and helps minimize further absorption
of the substance into the bloodstream. In
some cases of poisoning (for example,
corrosive poisons such as drain openers
that burn the esophagus), gastric lavage
is not performed because the tube that
must be inserted can cause further tissue
damage or puncture the esophagus.

(see page 132)

ASK YOUR DOCTOR
POISONING

Q My 4-year-old niece is coming
to stay for the weekend. I don't
think she can reach the medicine
cabinet, but I am worried. Which
medications should I lock away?

A Don't take a chance; you should
put all medications – both
prescription and over-the-counter
drugs – in a locked cabinet while your
niece is visiting. Remember to store
your household cleaning and gardening products out of her reach too.

Q A child in my neighborhood
almost died as a result of aspirin poisoning. If this can happen,
why is aspirin so easy to obtain?

A Aspirin is a safe drug if you
always follow the dosage instructions on the label. Do not give
aspirin to a child or teenager unless
you consult your doctor. Children
who get ahold of aspirin tablets usually spit them out because of their
bitter taste. If a child swallows a large
number of aspirin tablets, a potentially fatal chemical imbalance can
occur; get medical help immediately.

Q I have heard that if a child
swallows a battery it can corrode his or her stomach. Is this true
of used as well as new batteries?

A Yes. Any battery may be dangerous if swallowed because
stomach acid can corrode the metal
covering, releasing battery acid. Also,
some battery coverings are made of
lead, which poses a serious danger if
the lead covering is dissolved. If your
child swallows a battery, take him or
her to the nearest hospital emergency
department immediately. Keep batteries and items that contain batteries
out of the reach of children.

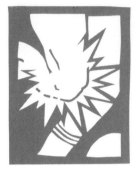

SPORTS INJURIES

REGULAR EXERCISE plays a key role in maintaining your physical fitness and health, but you can be injured during sports activities. For example, basketball injuries account for more than 600,000 hospital visits each year. The temperature of your environment influences your body's response to exercise and can lead to life-threatening conditions. In hot weather, restrict any strenuous exercise to the coolest hours of early morning or evening.

Most sports and recreational injuries are minor, such as bruises and strained or sprained muscles or ligaments. Many of these injuries are caused by overuse or overexertion rather than by an external force. Good physical conditioning, using proper safety equipment, and doing adequate warm-up and cool-down exercises can help reduce your risk of injury during sports activities.

Sports injuries
The incidence of specific injuries varies from sport to sport. For example, fractures occur more often in football than in basketball, while strains and sprains are more common injuries in basketball than in football.

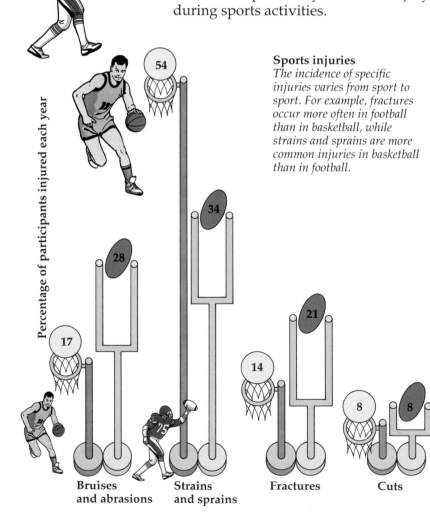

Percentage of participants injured each year

54
34
28
21
17
14
8
8

Bruises and abrasions · Strains and sprains · Fractures · Cuts

FIRST AID FOR MUSCLE AND JOINT INJURIES

First aid for muscle and joint injuries includes rest, ice, compression, and elevation (known as RICE).

REST the injured part of the body to reduce bleeding from damaged blood vessels in an injured muscle, to minimize the risk of further damage, and to allow time for tissues to heal.

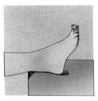

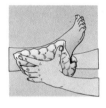

ICE relieves pain and limits swelling. Apply a cold pack for up to 10 minutes at a time (or until the area becomes numb or the skin turns red) every few hours for the first 2 days.

COMPRESSION limits bleeding and swelling. Wear a compression bandage around (and extending above and below) the injured area for at least 2 days. Loosen the bandage if it restricts blood flow.

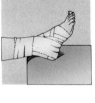

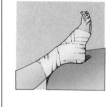

ELEVATION of the injured muscle or joint reduces swelling and bleeding. Keep the injured arm or leg raised above the level of the heart as much as possible.

REMOVING A HELMET

Do not remove a helmet from a person who may have a neck injury or is unconscious; you may cause more damage. Get medical help immediately. Remove the helmet only if the person is having difficulty or stops breathing. Face guards on some helmets may be removed without risking further injury caused by removing the helmet.

1 Call for medical help immediately. Place your hands on each side of the helmet, with your fingers on the person's lower jaw, to immobilize the head.

2 Another person should immobilize the head from below by applying pressure to the jaw using the thumb and index fingers of one hand while the other hand applies pressure at the base of the skull (shown at right).

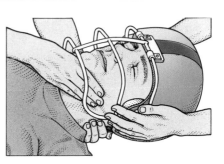

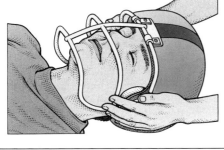

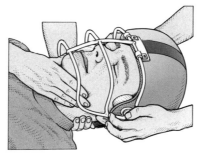

3 Keeping the head immobilized, spread the sides of the helmet and gently remove it.

4 You should keep the head immobilized from above by placing your hands on both sides of the person's head, with your palms over the ears (below). Start artificial ventilation (see page 47).

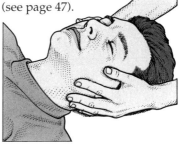

DISLOCATED JOINTS

A fall or strong force against a bone can displace the end of a bone from a joint. A dislocated joint appears misshapen and is tender and painful if moved. Never attempt to put a dislocated bone back into place; moving the bone may damage nerves and blood vessels. Immobilize the joint and see a doctor immediately.

STRAINS, SPRAINS, AND TEARS

Excessive stretching of a muscle can overstretch or tear some of the muscle fibers – injuries called muscle strains or pulled muscles. Overstretching that tears a large number of the muscle fibers is called a muscle tear. Bleeding inside an injured muscle causes pain, tenderness, swelling, and bruising. Overstretching may also tear a tendon or break off a piece of the bone to which the tendon is attached (see BASEBALL FINGER on page 84).

If the fibers of ligaments (which hold bones together) are overstretched and partially torn, the injury is called a sprain. Simply overstretching a ligament is called a strain; if many or all of the ligament fibers have been torn, the injury is called a tear. Symptoms of ligament injuries include pain made worse by moving the affected joint and tenderness, swelling, and instability of the joint.

Neck injuries

In contact sports, sudden forward-and-backward snapping motion of the neck can damage ligaments or muscles in the cervical (neck) region of the spine. Cervical strain or sprain injuries are characterized by discomfort and pain that radiates from the neck to the head or into the shoulders. Vertebrae in the neck may also be damaged in a person who has a cervical sprain or strain injury. If you suspect a person has a neck injury, immobilize the head and neck immediately (see page 73). Do not remove a helmet unless absolutely necessary (see above).

WARNING

Although regular exercise is associated with a substantially lower risk of a heart attack, strenuous physical activity may increase the risk of sudden death from cardiac arrest in people who may have heart disease. Consult your doctor before beginning a new exercise program.

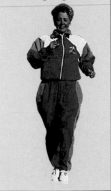

EFFECTS OF EXTREME TEMPERATURES

Your body systems work most efficiently when your body temperature is between 97 and 99°F. An area in your brain (called the hypothalamus) monitors body temperature and activates mechanisms (such as shivering or sweating) to compensate for changes. Exposure to extreme temperatures can cause failure of these temperature-regulating mechanisms.

Heat exhaustion

Strenuous physical activity in hot weather can cause heat exhaustion. Dizziness, nausea, fatigue, and muscle cramps are symptoms of heat exhaustion. Muscle cramps are caused by the loss of salt and fluid from the body as a result of very heavy sweating. If symptoms of heat exhaustion develop, lie down and rest in the shade. Drink cool water and place a cool, wet cloth on your forehead. If heat exhaustion is not treated promptly, it may progress to a more dangerous condition called heat stroke.

Heat stroke

Heat stroke is a life-threatening condition that develops if the body cannot cool itself effectively when exposed to extremely hot temperatures. People taking certain types of medication (such as antihistamines and some antidepressants) may be at increased risk of heat stroke (see WARNING on page 103). Heat stroke is often preceded by heat exhaustion. With the onset of heat stroke, sweating diminishes and the skin becomes flushed, hot, and usually dry. Body temperature often increases to 104 to 106°F. Without immediate first-aid treatment (see below), a victim of heat stroke may quickly lose consciousness and die.

Sunburn

Most cases of sunburn are mild, with some redness and tenderness. Prolonged exposure to the sun can lead to deeper burns on the skin, producing blisters and inflammation. Run cold water on sunburned skin. Seek medical attention for a severe sunburn; do not break blisters, rub the skin, or apply ointments.

SNOW-BLINDNESS

Prolonged exposure to the ultraviolet rays of the sun reflected by snow can damage the cornea (the transparent front part of the eye) and cause temporary loss of vision. Snowblindness causes the eyes to become red, painful, and sensitive to light. Although snowblindness is usually not serious, have your eyes checked by an ophthalmologist (eye doctor). Goggles with ultraviolet-filtering lenses help protect your eyes from snowblindness.

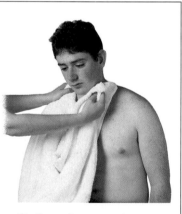

FIRST AID FOR HEAT STROKE

The most critical objective of first aid for heat stroke is to lower the body temperature as quickly as possible. Follow the first-aid guidelines given below.

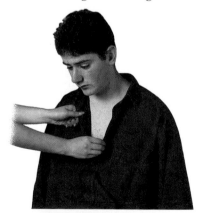

1 Call for medical help immediately. Move the person into the shade or to a cooler place and remove his or her clothing.

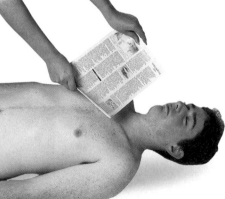

2 Apply moist, cool towels or cold packs (putting a cloth between the cold pack and the skin) or spray cold water from a hose onto the person. Fan the person, using a magazine or an electric fan.

3 Once the person's body temperature has fallen to about 101°F, dry off the person to prevent a chill. Check the person's temperature frequently; if his or her body temperature begins to rise again, repeat the cooling process until medical help arrives.

Frostbite

Frostbite occurs when parts of the body are exposed to very cold temperatures and freeze. It is caused by ice crystals forming in body tissues, which restricts blood flow to these tissues (see below).

While outside, cover frostbitten skin with extra clothing or a blanket. Do not rub the frostbitten area. Get the person inside and put the frostbitten part in warm water (about 100°F) or wrap the frostbitten area in blankets. Do not use hot-water bottles or heating pads because the skin may burn before sensation returns. Stop the warming process when the skin becomes pink or sensation returns. See a doctor promptly. If there is any possibility of the affected area refreezing, do not start the warming process before you can get medical help – simply keep the affected area covered.

Hypothermia

Hypothermia is chilling of the entire body to or below 95°F. Hypothermia may be caused by immersion in frigid water, prolonged exposure to extremely cold weather, or wearing damp clothing in very cold conditions. Hypothermia may cause shivering, numbness, drowsiness, muscle weakness, and low body temperature. In severe cases, breathing becomes slow and shallow and the person may become unconscious. First-aid instructions are given at right.

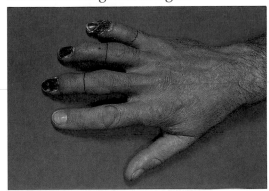

Symptoms of frostbite
In the early stages, frostbitten skin is painful and red. Pain disappears as feeling in the area is lost. The skin turns white or grayish yellow and blisters form. In severe cases, the skin may die, turning black.

FIRST AID FOR HYPOTHERMIA

Severe hypothermia can be life-threatening and requires prompt medical attention. If hypothermia is suspected, call for medical help immediately and start the first-aid warming process described here.

1 Maintain an open airway and restore breathing if necessary (see page 47).

2 Bring the person into a warm room as quickly as possible. Remove all wet clothes and wrap the person in dry towels or blankets.

3 (Not shown.) If the person is conscious, give him or her warm fluids, such as soup or broth. You should never give alcoholic beverages to a victim of hypothermia because alcohol opens up the blood vessels and causes more loss of body heat.

4 If the person cannot be moved, cover him or her with a blanket and call for medical help immediately. Lie close to the person to help warm him or her with your own body heat.

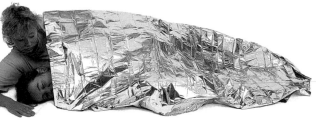

WARNING

You are more susceptible to extreme heat if you are very young or very old, overweight, or have a chronic illness. You are at increased risk from harmful effects of extreme cold if you are very old or very young, are wearing wet clothing, have wounds or fractures, have diseases that reduce the body's heat production, take certain medications (such as tranquilizers), smoke, or drink alcoholic beverages.

ENJOYING SPORTS SAFELY IN EXTREME HEAT OR COLD

Exposure to extreme heat or cold can stress the body's temperature-regulating mechanism and may result in mild discomfort or, in some cases, medical emergencies.

KEEPING COOL IN THE HEAT

Increased heat loss from the skin
The body loses heat as blood flows close to the surface of the skin. In hot weather, the blood vessels in the skin dilate (become wider), blood flow increases, and more heat is lost. Warm skin appears red because of the increased blood flow.

Sweating
Hot weather stimulates the production of moisture from sweat glands in the skin. The evaporation of this moisture has a cooling effect on the body. The efficiency of sweating as a way for your body to lose heat is reduced in humid weather because less evaporation takes place.

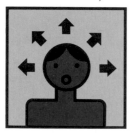

Heat is lost from the skin

Heat is received from the sun

Heat is received from the air

Heat is lost through sweating

Heat is generated by muscle activity and body metabolism

Heat is received from the ground

Overheating
In very hot, humid weather, when heat loss from sweating is decreased, your body may overheat as you receive more heat from the environment and generate more heat by physical activity than your body is able to lose.

Preventing heat exhaustion
Strenuous physical activity in hot weather can lead to dizziness, nausea, and fatigue – a condition called heat exhaustion. Do not overexert yourself. Wear lightweight, loose-fitting clothing and drink plenty of fluids.

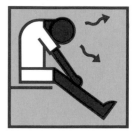

Preventing heat stroke
Be alert to the symptoms of heat exhaustion because heat stroke may soon follow. Heat stroke occurs when the body is dangerously overheated in hot, humid weather.

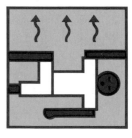

Preventing sunburn
Avoid the sun in the middle of the day, when ultraviolet rays are strongest. When in the sun, protect your skin with sunscreen (factor 15 or higher) or with clothing and a wide-brimmed hat.

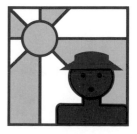

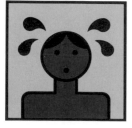

KEEPING WARM IN THE COLD

Reduced heat loss from the skin
In cold weather, blood vessels constrict (become narrower), conserving heat by reducing the blood flow to the skin. This reduced blood flow makes the skin appear more pale than usual.

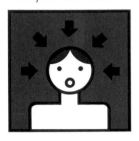

Shivering
To warm up in response to a drop in body temperature, you may begin shivering, which is a series of rapid, involuntary contractions and relaxations of the muscles. This muscle activity produces body heat.

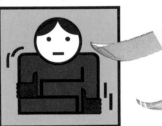

Heat is generated by muscle activity

Heat is lost from the skin

Heat is lost from the lungs in the breath

Body heat is partially retained by warm clothing

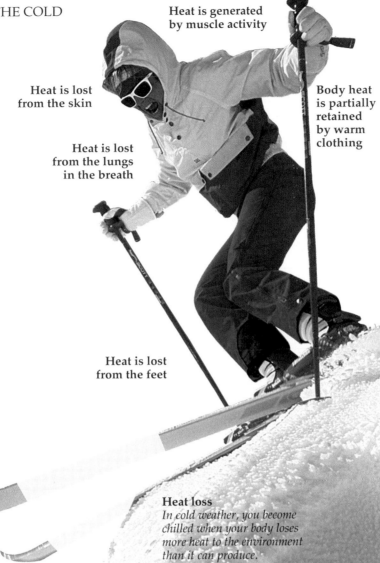

Heat is lost from the feet

Heat loss
In cold weather, you become chilled when your body loses more heat to the environment than it can produce.

Preventing frostbite
Frostbite is caused by extreme cold. Your nose, ears, fingers, and toes are most susceptible. Tie a scarf over your mouth and nose and wear thermal socks and gloves and a hat that covers your ears.

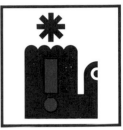

Preventing hypothermia
Hypothermia is severe chilling of the body. Avoid prolonged exposure to extreme cold, and do not swim in frigid water. In cold weather, wear layers of warm clothes – so skin moisture can evaporate – and change clothes if they get wet.

ALTITUDE SICKNESS

Altitude sickness can affect anyone who ascends too rapidly to heights above 8,000 feet. Altitude sickness is caused by the reduced oxygen levels at high altitudes. The lungs must work harder and the body's chemistry changes. Most cases of altitude sickness are mild, causing headache, nausea, and dizziness. In severe cases, fluid may escape from the blood vessels and build up in the lungs (called pulmonary edema), leading to severe breathlessness. If fluid builds up in the brain, symptoms may include hallucinations, seizures, and coma.

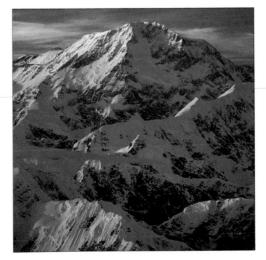

Preventing and treating altitude sickness
Gradual acclimatization (ascending over a period of days) and taking the drug acetazolamide may help prevent altitude sickness. Once altitude sickness occurs, the person must be brought down to a lower altitude as soon as possible. People with severe altitude sickness must be taken to a hospital immediately. Any delay could result in brain damage or death.

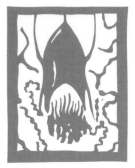

DROWNING AND WATER-SPORTS INJURIES

ALTHOUGH THE NUMBER of deaths by drowning has decreased by 33 percent since 1979, drowning is the third leading cause of accidental death, accounting for about 4,500 deaths each year. In addition, at least 70,000 people narrowly escape drowning. Among adults, alcohol intoxication is a factor in almost half of all drownings. When enjoying water sports, be aware of the dangers and take safety precautions to reduce your risk of injury.

Many water-related accidents can be prevented. Guidelines on how to enjoy a variety of water activities safely are given on page 32. You can greatly reduce your risk of drowning by never going swimming alone and by always swimming in areas that are supervised by lifeguards. Never overestimate your swimming abilities. Read all posted warning signs when you are swimming at the beach; waters with a strong undertow or fast currents are very dangerous, even for a strong, experienced swimmer. Safety tips on how you can help prevent drowning in backyard swimming pools are given on page 22.

RISK FACTORS

The highest incidence of death caused by drowning occurs during the summer, when we enjoy many leisure-time activities outdoors. For children and young adults aged 1 through 24, drowning is the second leading cause of death. Although the death rate for drownings among all age-groups has decreased, young children remain at extremely high risk. Toddlers are unsteady on their feet and can easily fall into a pool or off a river bank; these little ones can drown in only an inch or two of water.

Number of drownings by age
In 1989, the highest number of drownings occurred among adults aged 25 to 44 years, accounting for more than one fourth of all drownings. The 15- to 24-year-old age-group had the second highest number of drownings.

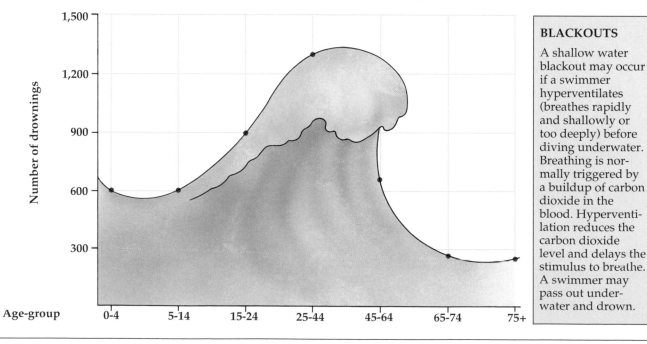

BLACKOUTS

A shallow water blackout may occur if a swimmer hyperventilates (breathes rapidly and shallowly or too deeply) before diving underwater. Breathing is normally triggered by a buildup of carbon dioxide in the blood. Hyperventilation reduces the carbon dioxide level and delays the stimulus to breathe. A swimmer may pass out underwater and drown.

DROWNING

Death by drowning is caused by suffocation, which occurs when a person lacks oxygen because he or she is unable to breathe. Suffocation may occur as a result of a reflex in which the vocal cords go into spasm (prolonged, strong contraction) and obstruct the airway (called dry drowning), or as a result of water being inhaled into the airway and lungs (called wet drowning).

Suffocation occurs after only a few minutes if a person is totally immersed in water. A person may be totally submerged for several minutes before the brain becomes dangerously deprived of oxygen; once this occurs, brain tissues begin to die within 2 or 3 minutes.

Water temperature is a significant factor in drowning. A person immersed in water loses body heat up to 27 times faster than in air that is the same temperature. Although wet clothes do not create warmth for a person who has fallen into cold water, the clothes insulate the body and reduce heat loss, delaying the onset of hypothermia (see page 103).

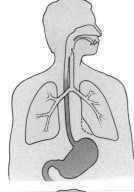

Wet drowning
Four fifths of the deaths caused by drowning are the result of wet drowning. In wet drowning, water is inhaled into the airway and lungs (left) as the person tries to breathe, causing suffocation.

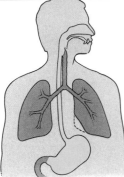

Dry drowning
Victims of dry drowning have a reflex of the vocal cords that closes the airway when water threatens to enter it, diverting the water away from the lungs and into the stomach (left). This reflex prevents breathing and causes suffocation.

SELF-HELP IN OPEN WATER

If you fall into open water without a life jacket, try to remain calm – do not panic. Do not thrash around in the water – movement increases the amount of body heat lost by dispersing the warmed water that is immediately surrounding your body. The following instructions will help you float until rescuers arrive.

Reduce heat loss
Reduce the amount of body heat lost in cold water by assuming a fetal position.

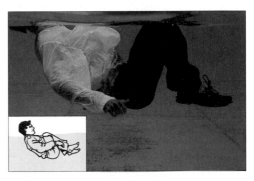

Making a float
Clothing can be used in an emergency as a temporary flotation device. Keep your arms in the sleeves of your shirt or jacket and pull the back of the clothing up and over your head (left). "Catch" a pocket of air and hold the bottom of the clothing under the water (below). Refill the air pocket at frequent intervals.

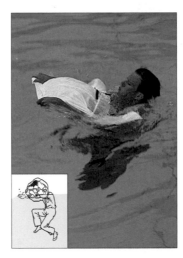

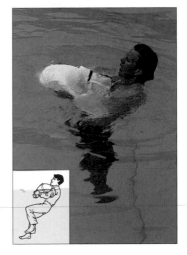

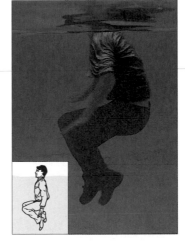

Treading water
Treading water enables you to keep your head above the water and requires less energy than swimming. You will tire easily if you try to swim against strong water currents.

HOW TO RESCUE A DROWNING PERSON

Most drownings occur in unsupervised areas. When attempting to rescue a drowning person, always keep your own safety in mind; stay calm and do not overestimate your strength. A drowning person can drag you down under the water.

If the person is not breathing:
Start mouth-to-mouth resuscitation (see page 47) as soon as you are able to support the person's body – either in a boat or in shallow water. When you get the person out of the water, lay the person on his or her back, continue mouth-to-mouth resuscitation, and begin cardiopulmonary resuscitation, if necessary.

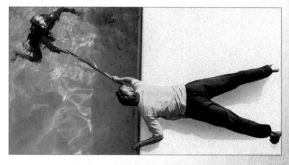

Rescuing someone within reach
More than half of all inland drownings occur within 9 feet of safety. If the drowning person is within your reach, lie down; give the person your hand or foot to grasp or reach out with a stick, pole, or life preserver; and pull the person to safety (above). If you are unable to reach a drowning person, row a boat out to the person (see below right).

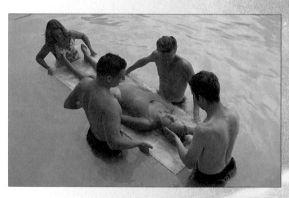

Rescuing a person with a neck or back injury
To rescue a diver or surfer with a suspected neck or back injury, place a board (such as a surfboard) under the person's head and back while he or she is still in the water. The board will help prevent movement that could further damage the neck, back, or spinal cord. (The board should extend from the head to the buttocks.) Lift the person out of the water on the board.

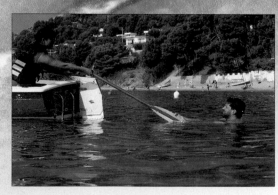

Boat rescue
Row out to the drowning person. Reach out to the person with an oar and pull him or her toward the boat. The person should hold on to the back of the boat while being rowed to shore. If this is not possible, pull the person carefully into the boat.

HOW TO MAKE A SWIMMING RESCUE

If you are unable to reach a drowning person from the side of a pool or from the shore and a boat is not available, swim out to the person. If possible, you should be secured by a rope to the shore, particularly if there is a strong water current or if the person is panicking. You should not attempt a swimming rescue unless you have learned and practiced lifesaving techniques (preferably from a Red Cross lifesaving course).

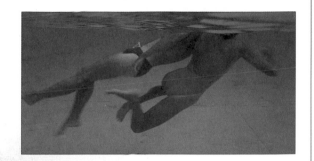

1 If the person panics, attempt to calm the person before making physical contact; otherwise he or she may struggle. Approach the person from behind and place one of your arms under the person's armpit. Do sidestrokes with your other arm and use a backstroke-type kick to tow the person to safety. Be sure to keep the person's head above the water.

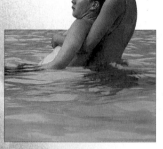

2 Check frequently to see that the person continues to breathe. If breathing stops, give mouth-to-mouth resuscitation as soon as possible (see page 47). Pull the person ashore. If a neck or back injury is suspected (see page 108), use a board to lift the person from the water.

4 If the person is breathing, place the person on his or her side so that fluids can drain from the person's mouth. Keep the person comfortably warm by covering him or her with a blanket or towel. Do not give food or water. If necessary, treat the person for shock (see page 57).

3 Once ashore, call for medical help immediately. Watch the person to make sure that he or she continues to breathe on his or her own. If breathing stops, give mouth-to-mouth resuscitation. If there is no heartbeat, start cardiopulmonary resuscitation immediately.

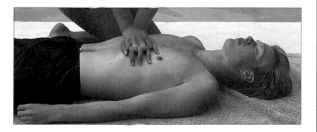

NEAR DROWNING

Young children have been resuscitated after prolonged immersion in water – called near drowning. Such miraculous recoveries generally occur when the child is very young and the water is very cold. Evidence suggests that a child who falls into cold water may stop breathing as a protective reflex, before water enters the lungs. A second reflex (called the diving reflex) then slows the heartbeat and conserves the oxygen in the blood for the heart and brain. The rapid cooling of a child's body by the cold water reduces his or her oxygen requirements so that a child may be able to survive without oxygen for extended periods of time. Adults are less likely to survive such immersions in cold water because they no longer have a diving reflex.

WATER-SPORTS INJURIES

Waterskiing accidents are often the result of careless driving of a speedboat. When pulling a waterskier, there should always be at least two people in the boat – one to drive and the other to watch the skier. If the skier falls, shout to the skier to make sure he or she is all right. If the person has been injured, watch him or her closely until he or she can be pulled from the water. Never leave a tow bar trailing in the water; it may cause serious injuries when the boat is traveling at a high speed.

Life jackets
You should always wear a life jacket when boating or enjoying other water sports. Nine out of 10 drownings involve occupants of small boats. In open water or in water with strong currents, even excellent swimmers can drown.

Drivers of speedboats should continuously scan the water for swimmers because the sharp blades of a boat's propeller can cause severe injuries.

Diving injuries

Always check the water depth before diving. Diving into shallow water causes hundreds of spinal injuries every year, many resulting in permanent paralysis (loss of movement). High diving can cause back strains and neck injuries if entry into the water is not straight.

A common and serious hazard of scuba diving is decompression sickness (also called "the bends"). Decompression sickness may cause severe abdominal or chest pain, blood in the urine, or severe pain in bones, muscles, and joints. Symptoms may also include paralysis or other disturbances of the nervous system that may indicate a stroke. A diver with decompression sickness needs immediate medical treatment.

What causes decompression sickness?
As a diver descends, the pressure of water on the body increases. Under this increasing pressure, nitrogen from the diver's air supply dissolves rapidly into body tissues. When the diver ascends too quickly, pressure falls and the nitrogen is rapidly released from the tissues, forming bubbles that block circulation in the blood vessels and causing symptoms.

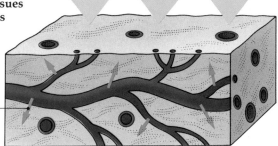

During descent, pressure on body tissues increases

Nitrogen is dissolved into tissues at a higher rate

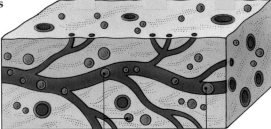

During ascent, pressure on body tissues decreases

If ascent is too rapid, released nitrogen forms bubbles in tissues and blood vessels

Blood vessel blocked by nitrogen bubble

CASE HISTORY
DRINKING AND SWIMMING

SCOTT AND HIS CLASSMATES had been celebrating their high school graduation by drinking beer down by the lake. As Scott and his friends walked along the lake, one of the boys dared him to swim across. Scott considered himself a good swimmer so he jumped into the water.

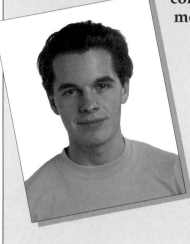

PERSONAL DETAILS
Name Scott Foster
Age 18
Occupation Student
Family Scott has two younger brothers and a sister in college.

THE INCIDENT
Scott starts swimming and he is confident he can easily swim to the other side of the lake. Only a few feet from the shore, he swallows some water and starts choking. He begins struggling to stay afloat.

FIRST AID
Scott's friends have been drinking and think Scott is kidding around, pretending to be drowning. A man, Al Horowicz, out walking his dog sees Scott struggling in the water and rushes over to the edge of the lake. Al quickly finds a long tree branch, lies down on the shore, and holds the branch out to Scott. Scott is able to grab the branch, and Al pulls him to the shore.

Once ashore, Al yells to another passerby to call an ambulance. He then checks Scott's airway and sees that he is breathing. To prevent Scott from choking on fluids or vomit, Al rolls Scott onto his side. He tells a friend of Scott's to take off his jacket and cover Scott to keep him warm, and tells one of the other boys to call Scott's parents.

AT THE HOSPITAL
The doctor in the emergency department examines Scott. He tells Scott that he finds no immediate problems but would like to keep him in the hospital for observation. The doctor explains to Scott that he may have inhaled water that contained foreign particles, which could lead to inflammation of his lungs. This condition, called aspiration pneumonia, may cause breathing difficulties. The doctor comes out to the waiting room and reassures Scott's parents that he is going to be okay. Scott's parents go into the emergency department to see Scott; as they are talking to him they smell alcohol on his breath. Scott is released from the hospital after 36 hours.

THE OUTCOME
Scott tells his parents that he doesn't remember much about what happened. His parents tell him that they are very upset and disappointed that Scott acted so irresponsibly. They remind him of the dangers of drinking alcohol before swimming because of the detrimental effects that alcohol has on reaction time, hand-eye coordination, balance, and muscle strength. Scott assures his parents that he has learned a very frightening lesson and that he will never drink and swim again.

Safely on shore
Al places Scott on his side to make sure that fluids can drain out of Scott's mouth.

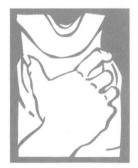

BREATHING EMERGENCIES

BREATHING EMERGENCIES occur when a person's airway is blocked or partially obstructed. The efficiency of the airway can be reduced as a result of asthma and other respiratory conditions. Obstruction of the airway may have a sudden cause, such as a foreign object caught in the throat or strangulation. An allergic reaction or burns may cause the airway to become obstructed as a result of swelling of the soft tissues in the airway.

Breathing emergencies always require immediate action – any interruption of oxygen to the brain for more than a few minutes may lead to brain damage or death. Being able to recognize the signs and symptoms of breathing difficulties and knowing how to give artificial ventilation may help save a person's life.

ASTHMA

Asthma is a condition in which the bronchioles (the small airways in the lungs) become constricted (narrowed), causing breathlessness that is often accompanied by a feeling of tightness of the chest and

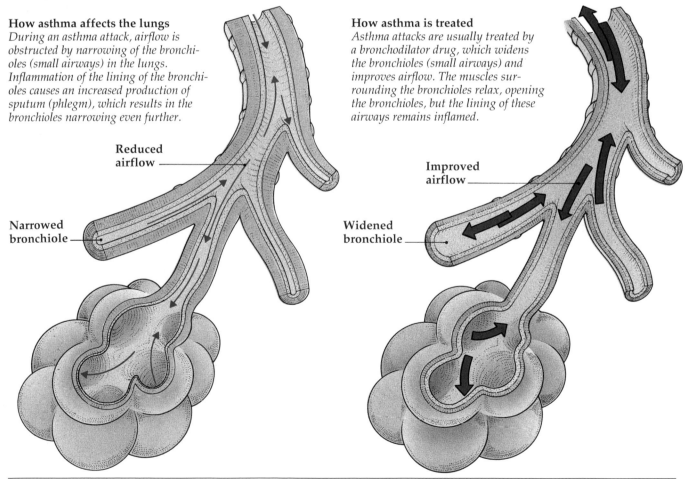

How asthma affects the lungs
During an asthma attack, airflow is obstructed by narrowing of the bronchioles (small airways) in the lungs. Inflammation of the lining of the bronchioles causes an increased production of sputum (phlegm), which results in the bronchioles narrowing even further.

Reduced airflow

Narrowed bronchiole

How asthma is treated
Asthma attacks are usually treated by a bronchodilator drug, which widens the bronchioles (small airways) and improves airflow. The muscles surrounding the bronchioles relax, opening the bronchioles, but the lining of these airways remains inflamed.

Improved airflow

Widened bronchiole

wheezing. This condition frequently starts in childhood and tends to clear up or become less severe in early adulthood. The cause of asthma attacks in most people is often an external substance that has been inhaled or eaten. For example, an allergy to grasses, pollens, molds, some food additives, and some drugs can trigger an asthma attack. Asthma may also be caused by infections of the respiratory tract, such as pneumonia or bronchitis. Some asthma attacks have no apparent cause.

During a severe asthma attack, breathing becomes increasingly difficult and is accompanied by sweating and rapid heartbeat. The person may be unable to speak. In a very severe asthma attack, the low amount of oxygen in the blood may lead to cyanosis (blue discoloration of the lips and tissues under the nails). Some attacks can be fatal.

Most asthma attacks can be controlled by drugs – called bronchodilators – that widen (dilate) the bronchioles. In some cases, the attack may be so severe that it requires emergency medical treatment such as the administration of oxygen and corticosteroid drug therapy. In very severe cases, breathing is assisted by inserting a tube down the throat into the trachea (the windpipe). A ventilator (a machine that forces oxygen under pressure into the lungs) may be connected to the tube to maintain breathing.

PULMONARY EDEMA

Pulmonary edema is a dangerous condition in which fluid accumulates in the tissues of the lungs. The most common cause of pulmonary edema is heart failure, in which the heart is unable to pump out blood as fast as blood is returned from the lungs (see above right). Other causes include severe lung infections, inhalation of irritant gases, and altitude sickness (see page 105). Symptoms of pulmonary edema include breathlessness, coughing, sweating, and anxiety.

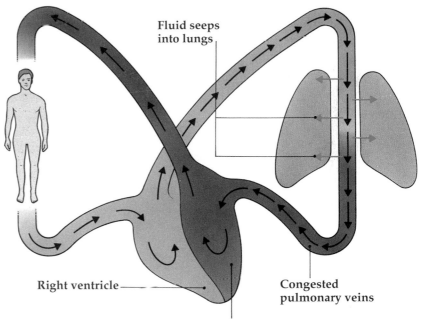

Fluid seeps into lungs

Right ventricle

Left ventricle

Congested pulmonary veins

Pulmonary edema requires treatment in a hospital, where the person is given oxygen to reduce breathlessness and a diuretic drug to draw fluid out of the lungs. People with pulmonary edema caused by altitude sickness must be moved to a lower altitude immediately.

CROUP

Croup is the name for a group of symptoms caused by a variety of respiratory conditions in infants and young children. Croup is usually caused by a viral infection and tends to occur most frequently in the fall and winter. Often the child has a mild cold before the attack.

Symptoms may include difficulty breathing, wheezing or grunting when inhaling, hoarseness, a barklike cough, slight fever, and restlessness. Attacks of croup often occur after the child has gone to bed. Most attacks are mild and pass quickly. Comfort the child if he or she becomes frightened; once the child calms down, he or she may be able to breathe more easily. Placing a vaporizer in the child's room or taking the child into a steam-filled bathroom may help the child breathe. If the child is struggling to breathe or turns blue, call an ambulance.

Heart failure and pulmonary edema
Pulmonary edema caused by heart failure occurs when the left side of the heart is unable to efficiently pump out blood. As a result, the veins that carry oxygen-rich blood from the lungs to the heart become congested with blood. As the congestion in the veins from the lungs increases, this pressure causes fluid to collect in the lungs, making it much more difficult for oxygen to pass through the lung tissues and get into the bloodstream.

CHOKING

Obstruction of the upper part of the airway, commonly called choking (see below), occurs when the airway is partially or totally obstructed by an object. Choking is the sixth most common cause of accidental death. It is especially common in children under 4 years old who have put objects in their mouths. An object stuck in the throat may cause the child's voice to sound strained or strange. Call an ambulance. Do not interfere with the child's attempts to cough out the object and do not stick your fingers down his or her throat. First aid for choking is discussed in THE HEIMLICH MANEUVER on page 52. A cricothyrotomy may be necessary (see right).

Signs of choking
A person who is choking starts to gasp or breathe noisily and involuntarily grasps at his or her throat. Breathing becomes difficult and may stop. If the airway is completely obstructed, the person will become unconscious if first aid is not given promptly (see page 52).

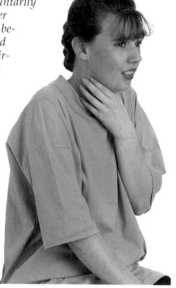

SUFFOCATION

Suffocation is a condition in which normal breathing is prevented, resulting in a lack of oxygen to the lungs. External obstruction of the mouth and nose – for example, if a person has become accidentally buried in a mining or construction cave-in or if an infant is lying face

CRICOTHYROTOMY

If a person is having breathing difficulties caused by an object in the airway that cannot be dislodged (see THE HEIMLICH MANEUVER on page 52), an emergency procedure called a cricothyrotomy may be necessary to open the airway. Call for medical help immediately. A tracheostomy can be performed after a cricothyrotomy, if necessary. A tracheostomy is an operation (usually performed while the person is under general anesthesia in a hospital) in which an opening is made in the trachea (windpipe) and a tube is inserted to keep the airway open.

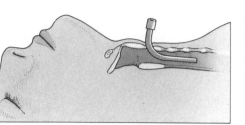

Performing a cricothyrotomy
To perform a cricothyrotomy, the trained rescuer or doctor makes an incision in the skin over the center front of the throat. A small incision is made through the cricothyroid membrane and a metal or plastic tube is inserted to keep the airway open until the object that is obstructing the airway can be removed.

down on a pillow and cannot move his or her head – may cause suffocation. Suffocation may be caused by inhaling poisonous gases (such as carbon monoxide) that interfere with the uptake of oxygen into the bloodstream. Symptoms of suffocation may include drowsiness, difficulty breathing, noisy breathing, frothing at the mouth, discoloration of the lips, seizures, loss of consciousness, coma, and death. First-aid treatment of suffocation is discussed below.

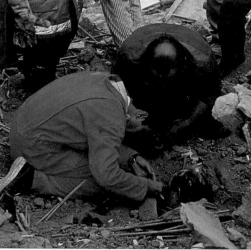

First aid for suffocation
Remove the obstructing object from the face and throat. If the cause is a poisonous gas, move the person into fresh air. If the person has been buried in an accident, try to clear off the dirt or debris down to the hips so that his or her chest can expand during breathing. Call an ambulance immediately, and give artificial ventilation, if necessary, until medical help arrives.

STRANGULATION

Strangulation with a cord or rope causes compression of the carotid arteries in the neck. This prevents blood from flowing to the brain, and the person loses consciousness. The pressure of the cord or rope may also squeeze the airway shut and block the flow of air to the lungs. Remove the rope or cord from the victim's neck immediately. If there is a knot, cut below it. Call for medical help immediately. A hanging victim may have a spinal injury (see page 72). If the person is unconscious, complete the ABCs (airway, breathing, and circulation) of resuscitation (see page 45).

EPIGLOTTITIS

Epiglottitis is a serious and sometimes fatal infection of the epiglottis (the flap of tissue at the back of the throat that closes off the windpipe during swallowing). The epiglottis becomes inflamed and swollen, obstructing the airway. Symptoms may include fever, loss of voice, painful swallowing, drooling, difficulty breathing, and a forward thrusting of the jaw (to keep the airway open). A person who has epiglottitis requires immediate treatment in the hospital. Treatment may include antibiotics, oxygen, and insertion of a tube down the windpipe to keep the airway open.

HYPERVENTILATION

Hyperventilation is rapid and shallow or abnormally deep breathing that is usually caused by anxiety. It may also occur as a result of uncontrolled diabetes mellitus, oxygen deficiency, kidney failure, and some lung disorders.

Hyperventilation causes an abnormal loss of carbon dioxide that leads to alkalosis (a disturbance in the body's acid-base balance) and a drop in the level of blood calcium. A person who is hyperventilating may have a feeling of tightness in the chest, awareness of the heartbeat, muscle spasms, numbness in the fingers and around the mouth, and dizziness. These symptoms add to the person's existing anxiety and he or she may experience narrowing of the field of vision and a feeling of impending doom.

Treating hyperventilation
Breathing in and out of a paper bag should be done only if you can be sure the hyperventilation is caused by anxiety and not by a serious medical condition. If you have any doubt as to the cause of the hyperventilation, call for medical help immediately.

ASK YOUR DOCTOR
BREATHING EMERGENCIES

Q My 4-year-old son has temper tantrums during which he holds his breath until his face turns blue. Could he suffocate doing this?

A No. Eventually your son's natural protective mechanisms will start him breathing again. This may not happen until he has lost consciousness for a few seconds. When your son loses consciousness, his throat and airway muscles will relax and he will start breathing.

Q I have read that the body is able to store oxygen. If this is the case, why is there so little time in which to rescue a person who is having trouble breathing?

A It is true that hemoglobin, the pigment contained in red blood cells, is able to store oxygen – but only temporarily. The amount of oxygen required by the body tissues is so great that in the absence of inhaled oxygen the stored oxygen is depleted in minutes. The brain may suffer irreversible damage after 4 to 10 minutes without oxygen.

Q Is there anything I can do if I have an asthma attack and I have forgotten my inhaler?

A If you don't have your inhaler with you during an asthma attack, sit down in a position that allows you to breathe as comfortably as possible and try to stay calm. If the attack lasts for more than a few minutes or is severe, call for medical help. To prevent such an occurrence, you may want to keep an inhaler at home, at work, and in the car. As with all medications, keep your inhaler out of the reach of children.

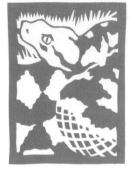

BITES AND STINGS

BITES AND STINGS ARE TYPES of puncture wounds. Animal and human bites can cause serious infection. Some animals inject venom (poison) under the skin when they bite or sting. Many bites and stings cause only redness and swelling around the site of the puncture, but a bite or sting can be life-threatening if the venom is extremely poisonous or if a person is allergic to the venom.

Most bites are from domestic animals – between 1 and 2 million people are bitten by dogs and cats every year. Poisonous snakes bite about 8,000 people every year. Stings are usually less serious than bites, causing only mild skin reactions. But some stings can be very dangerous; severe allergic reactions to insect stings cause more deaths per year than snakebites. Some venoms injected by bites and stings are more dangerous than others, causing symptoms that range from fever and vomiting to difficulty breathing, heart failure, and death.

TREATING BITES AND STINGS

Although most spiders produce venom, only a few species of spiders are harmful to humans. The two most dangerous spiders are the black widow and the brown recluse. Most insect stings require little treatment other than carefully washing the site of the sting. But stings can be life-threatening if a person has a severe allergic reaction to the venom. Stings from some marine animals are very dangerous and require immediate treatment.

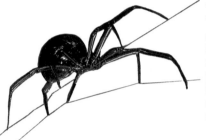

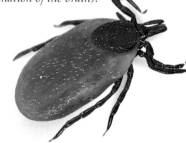

Tick bites
Ticks spread infectious organisms by attaching themselves to skin to feed on blood. An attached tick may not be noticed for hours; others cause irritation, pain, or bruising. Ticks can spread the bacterial infection Lyme disease and certain types of viral encephalitis (inflammation of the brain).

Black widow spider bites
A bite from a black widow spider may cause redness, pain, and swelling around the bite; profuse sweating; nausea and sometimes vomiting; stomach cramps; muscle cramps; a feeling of tightness in the chest; and difficulty breathing.

Treating tick bites
Using tweezers, grasp the tick at its head (see below) and pull it out slowly. Do not try to pull the tick out with your fingers, because the head may break away from the body and stay embedded in the skin. Clean the bite with rubbing alcohol or an antiseptic. If the tick head stays embedded, see your doctor immediately.

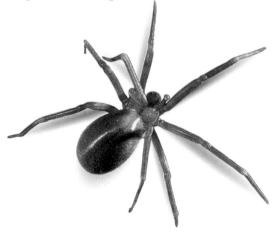

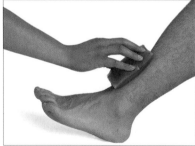

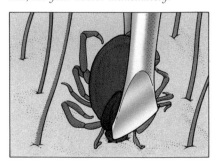

Brown recluse spider bites
A bite from a brown recluse spider produces a stinging sensation, followed by redness and the formation of blisters. If the bite is not treated quickly, pain becomes more severe; deep, irreversible tissue damage around the bite may lead to an open sore.

Treating spider bites
Keep the bitten area immobilized and lower than the person's heart. Place a cold pack on the bite and get medical help immediately. Maintain an open airway and restore breathing if necessary (see page 47). If you can do so safely, capture the spider for identification.

Insect stings

The most common stinging insects are honeybees, hornets, wasps, and fire ants. Symptoms of insect stings include pain, swelling, redness, itching, and burning. Some insects leave their stingers when they sting.

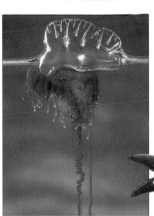

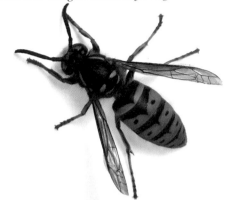

Treating insect stings

Remove a stinger by carefully scraping the skin with a clean knife or fingernail. Do not grasp the stinger to remove it; this may force more venom into the skin. Wash the area with soap and water and place a cold pack on the sting. Applying calamine lotion may relieve discomfort.

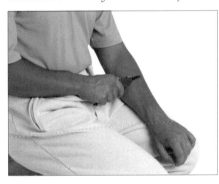

Marine-life stings

Stings from some forms of marine life, particularly the Portuguese man-of-war, are poisonous. Symptoms may include intense burning pain, reddening of the skin, muscle cramps, nausea, vomiting, difficulty breathing, and sometimes shock.

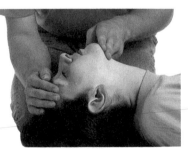

Treating marine-life stings

Wrap a cloth around your hands and remove attached tentacles. Pour large amounts of seawater over the sting and wash the area with rubbing alcohol or vinegar. Treat for shock if necessary (see page 57). Seek immediate medical help.

Scorpion stings

A scorpion sting may cause intense burning pain at the site of the sting, stomach pain, nausea and vomiting, numbness and tingling in the affected area, possible spasm of jaw muscles, shock, seizures, and sometimes coma.

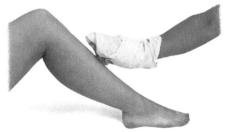

Treating scorpion stings

Keep the area of the sting lower than the person's heart. Place a cold pack on the sting and get medical help immediately. Treat for shock if necessary (see page 57). Maintain an open airway and restore breathing and circulation if necessary (see page 45).

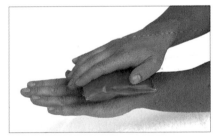

ANAPHYLACTIC SHOCK

Anaphylactic shock is a potentially life-threatening allergic reaction that can occur a few seconds to a couple of hours after an insect bite or sting. Symptoms may include severe swelling around the eyes or of the lips and tongue (as well as swelling at the site of the bite or sting), rash, coughing or wheezing, difficulty breathing, stomach cramps, nausea and vomiting, weakness, dizziness, and, possibly, unconsciousness. Call for medical help immediately and follow the first-aid instructions given at right.

1 Maintain an open airway and restore breathing and circulation if necessary (see page 45). Remove the stinger if there is one (see TREATING INSECT STINGS above).

2 Place a cold pack on the sting to prevent the spread of venom. Keep the person lying down unless he or she is short of breath; if so, let the person sit up. Treat for shock if necessary (see page 57).

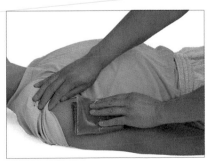

SNAKEBITES

Poisonous snakes include rattlesnakes (of which there are about 10 different species), water moccasins (also called cottonmouths), copperheads, and coral snakes. Rattlesnakes are found all over the country. Water moccasins and copperheads are found primarily in the southeast and central southern parts of the US. Coral snakes are found primarily in the southeast and southwest.

Characteristics of poisonous snakes
Rattlesnakes, water moccasins, and copperheads have triangular-shaped heads and are called pit vipers. These snakes can be recognized by deep pits between the eyes and nostrils. They also have slitlike eyes. Unlike the pit vipers, the coral snake has round eyes.

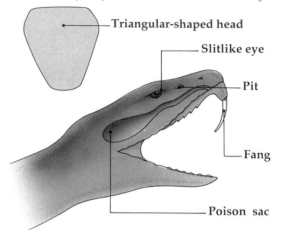

— Triangular-shaped head

— Slitlike eye

— Pit

— Fang

— Poison sac

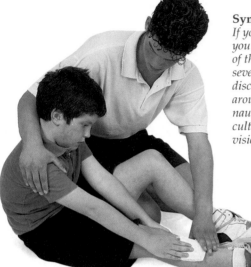

Symptoms of snakebites
If you are bitten by a snake, you may experience any or all of the following symptoms: severe pain, rapid swelling, discoloration of the skin around the bite, weakness, nausea and vomiting, difficulty breathing, blurred vision, seizures, and shock.

Water moccasin
Water moccasins have a distinctive white coloring inside the mouth. This snake lives in or near water.

Rattlesnake
Rattlesnakes have a set of rattles at the end of their tails that they vibrate when they are disturbed. Most rattlesnakes are pale brown; some have a diamond pattern or black bands on their body.

Coral snake
The coral snake is a member of the cobra family. Its markings consist of yellow, red, and black rings, with the yellow rings separating the red rings from the black. The coral snake has a black nose. These colors are mimicked by other nonpoisonous snakes, but in nonpoisonous snakes the red bands are bordered by the black bands.

Copperhead
A copperhead snake has red-brown (or dark brown) and light brown bands, with a copper colored head. It vibrates its tail when it is disturbed.

FIRST AID FOR SNAKEBITES

Immediate first aid for snakebites attempts to slow the spread of venom by restricting the flow of blood. Never put cold packs on a snakebite; tissue damage can result. First aid for poisonous snakebites (except the coral snake – see right) is explained below.

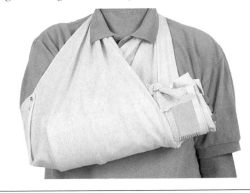

First aid for coral snake bites
If a person has been bitten by a coral snake, quickly wash the affected area. Immobilize a bitten arm or leg with a splint (see page 87). Do not tie off the bitten area or apply a cold pack. Keep the person sitting or lying still and get medical help immediately.

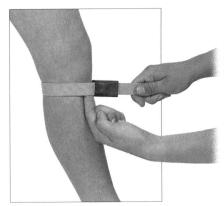

1 If the snakebite is on an arm or leg, place a light, constricting band (such as a belt) 2 to 4 inches above the bite. The band should not be so tight that it cuts off the circulation. You should feel a pulse below the level of the band and be able to slip your finger under the band with a little resistance. The wound should ooze.

2 If the area around the band begins to swell, remove the band and place it 2 to 4 inches above the first site. Do not remove the band completely. Wash the area thoroughly with soap and water. Immobilize a bitten arm or leg with a splint (see page 87).

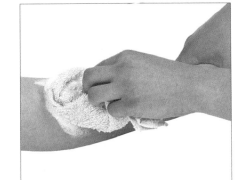

3 If you are only a short distance from a hospital, take the person there immediately. Otherwise, if you have a snakebite kit, use the blade provided; or sterilize a knife or razor blade. Make a cut $1/8$ to $1/4$ inch deep (and no longer than a $1/2$ inch) through each fang mark along the long axis of the limb; do not cut any deeper.

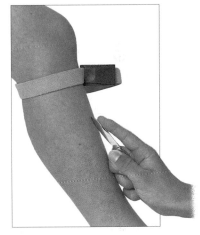

4 If you have suction cups from a snakebite kit, place them over the wound and draw out the body fluids (which contain venom); if suction cups are not available, use your mouth if it is free of cuts and sores. Do not swallow the venom; spit it out. Continue suction for 30 minutes or more and rinse your mouth out.

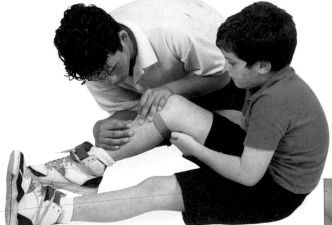

5 Cover the wound with a clean cloth or bandage. Do not let the person walk unless absolutely necessary. The person may have sips of water if he or she has no difficulty swallowing and is not nauseated, vomiting, or having seizures. Go to the nearest emergency department immediately; if possible, call ahead so antivenin (see right) can be obtained.

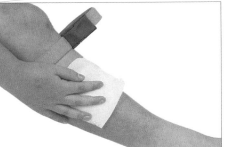

ANTIVENINS

Poisonous snakebites are usually treated with an injection of antivenin (a preparation that contains antibodies against the poison). Antivenins are available to treat bites by all pit vipers and by coral snakes. Almost all people with poisonous snakebites who receive prompt medical attention survive, with minimal aftereffects (such as tissue damage).

ASK YOUR DOCTOR
BITES AND STINGS

Q I am going camping with some friends and have been told that there are poisonous snakes in the area. What can we do to protect ourselves from snakebites?

A To avoid snakebites, wear long pants and boots, stay on cleared trails when hiking, use a stick to move large rocks or logs, don't sleep on the ground, and never disturb or try to kill a snake – move away from it slowly. Take a snakebite kit with you and learn the first-aid procedures before you go. If you are bitten, go to the nearest hospital emergency department.

Q My son is around animals when he plays outside. How can I tell if an animal has rabies?

A A rabid animal may appear disoriented, often foaming at the mouth. But some rabid animals appear normal. Teach your children never to feed or play with wild or strange animals. If you think an animal has rabies, call the police or local health department immediately.

Q My daughter was recently stung by a bee. She had a severe allergic reaction and was rushed to the hospital. The doctor in the emergency department said she should always carry a special emergency kit. What is in this kit?

A The emergency kit usually includes a syringe that contains epinephrine. This drug is injected immediately after a sting to reduce the severity of the allergic reaction. Other medications that may be useful to keep in the kit are antihistamine and corticosteroid drugs. Your family doctor can advise you on where you can obtain the kit and how to use it.

ANIMAL BITES

Bites by domestic pets and wild animals can become infected. They also carry the risk of tetanus and rabies. In the US, an estimated 10,000 people bitten by an animal receive antirabies treatment each year. But fewer than five people get rabies each year, a result of intensive vaccinations of dogs and prompt medical treatment of animal bites.

Clean an animal bite with soap and running water for 5 minutes or more. Cover the bite with a sterile bandage or clean cloth and see a doctor immediately. Antibiotics and injections to prevent tetanus and rabies may be given. A person who is bitten by an animal that may be rabid must be given a series of shots to build up the body's immunity in time to prevent the disease. Once symptoms appear, rabies is fatal (see below). If you think an animal has rabies, call the police or your local health department so the animal can be captured and observed for signs of rabies.

Rabies virus
The rabies virus (right) can be transmitted to humans by the saliva of infected animals. Transmission of rabies by domestic dogs is uncommon. Animals most likely to carry the rabies virus are skunks, bats, foxes, and raccoons.

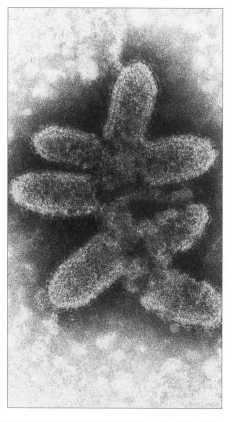

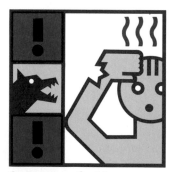

Symptoms of rabies
Symptoms may appear weeks or months after being bitten by a rabid animal. Initially, fever, headache, and loss of appetite occur, followed by restlessness, hyperactivity, disorientation, and seizures. Coma and death follow within days.

HUMAN BITES

Human bites that break the skin can cause serious infections from bacteria in the mouth that may enter the wound. Human bites are usually associated with higher rates of infection than animal bites. Clean the bite with soap and running water for 5 minutes or more. Do not apply antiseptics or anything else to the bite. Put a sterile bandage or clean cloth over the wound and get medical help immediately. Antibiotics are usually given to prevent infection; a tetanus booster shot is also given if needed.

CASE HISTORY
A HUNGRY RACCOON

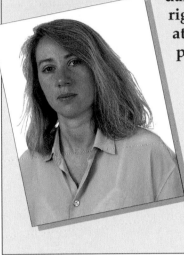

LATE ONE EVENING, Carrie went outside to put a bag of garbage into the trash cans alongside the garage. She noticed that one of the cans had tipped over and that the garbage had spilled into the yard. It was too dark to try to clean up the mess right away, but Carrie wanted to at least pick up the trash can and put the lid back on.

PERSONAL DETAILS
Name Carrie Slimski
Age 29
Occupation Office manager
Family Carrie is married with no children.

THE INCIDENT
Carrie reaches down to pick up the trash can that has tipped over. As she starts to bring the can upright, she hears a scuffling noise and a raccoon suddenly runs out from behind the can. Carrie feels a sharp pain in her right calf and she screams. Hearing Carrie's scream, her husband, Eric, runs out to see what happened. Eric helps Carrie back into the house to check her leg.

FIRST AID
Carrie's calf is bleeding from the bite and is starting to throb painfully. Eric gently but thoroughly cleans the wound with soap and water and covers it with a sterile gauze pad from their first-aid kit. He then drives Carrie to their local hospital emergency department.

AT THE HOSPITAL
At the emergency department, the doctor asks Carrie what happened. The doctor examines the bite on Carrie's leg, cleans it again to reduce the risk of infection, and bandages the wound. She explains to Carrie that, because of the risk that the raccoon was infected with the rabies virus, she is going to give her two injections (one at the site

Treating the wound
To help make sure that contaminating organisms are washed out of the raccoon bite, the doctor cleans the wound with soap and water and rinses it with sterile fluid. She then applies an antiseptic to help prevent infection and bandages the wound.

of the bite and one into the muscles in her buttocks) of antibodies to the rabies virus to prevent the disease from developing. The doctor tells Carrie that additional injections are necessary and asks her to come back in 3 days. She also gives Carrie a tetanus shot (since her last booster shot was more than 10 years ago) and prescribes antibiotics. The doctor recommends that Carrie keep her calf elevated as much as possible to help reduce the swelling.

THE OUTCOME
Carrie is able to go back to work in a few days. She returns to the hospital for the necessary injections over the next 3 months. Each time, the doctor examines Carrie to check for signs of rabies and makes sure the wound has not become infected. No signs of rabies develop.

CHAPTER FOUR

EMERGENCY MEDICAL CARE

INTRODUCTION

EMERGENCY
MEDICAL SERVICES

THE EMERGENCY
DEPARTMENT

NJURIES AND ILLNESS can occur suddenly and can be severe. In the past, society was not adequately prepared for medical emergencies and many people died before help could reach them. The first recorded mention of ambulances was in the 11th century. Prehospital emergency care started in the 1700s during the Napoleonic wars, when medical care in the field and evacuation by hot-air balloon occurred.

Until the 1960s, the main function of emergency services was to transport a person to a hospital as quickly as possible, providing little or no lifesaving care on the way. Today, in many communities, a closely coordinated network of emergency services for people with an injury or sudden illness is available 24 hours a day. The emergency medical services system includes a telephone number for calling a dispatcher to send an ambulance, the emergency medical technicians (EMTs) and ambulances, a communications system between EMTs and hospital personnel, and hospital emergency departments.

The emergency medical care provided by this system is organized into prehospital and hospital care. Nationally, the prehospital component consists of more than half a million EMTs working with about 35,000 ambulances and more than 600 aircraft. The

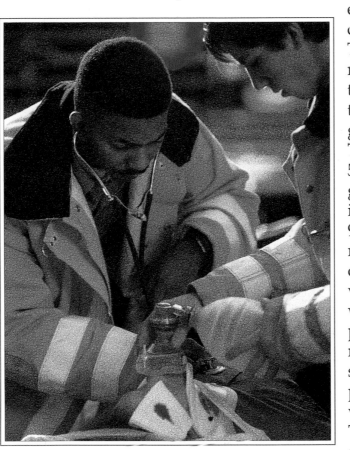

EMTs assess the condition of the person, remove the person from any danger, and provide emergency medical care. Until the person is transferred to the care of the doctors and nurses in the hospital emergency department, the EMTs maintain radio contact with medical personnel in a designated hospital. The EMTs communicate information on the patient's condition to these professionals, who direct the EMTs on the emergency medical care that is needed.

The second component of emergency treatment begins in the hospital emergency department. There are more than 5,000 hospital emergency departments in the US, staffed by 95,000 doctors and nurses. Emergency departments provide care to people with less serious problems (such as minor cuts and sprains) as well as to people who are severely ill or injured. To properly care for a large number of accident victims at one time, emergency department personnel use a system of categorizing and sorting patients according to the severity of their injuries. This system, known as triage, ensures that the patients most urgently in need of medical care are treated first. If a patient's life is in danger, he or she is treated immediately in the emergency department and may then be taken to the operating room or admitted to the hospital.

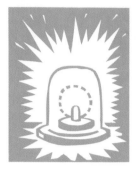

EMERGENCY MEDICAL SERVICES

A BOUT HALF the communities across the country use 911 to contact the emergency medical services (EMS) system; others have designated seven-digit emergency numbers. The primary goals of the EMS system are to provide medical care at the scene of an emergency and on the way to a hospital, rapid transportation to a hospital, and a hospital network that ensures a person receives the appropriate level of care for his or her injury or illness.

Emergency services personnel
Emergency medical services personnel include emergency medical technicians (EMTs), who treat the person at the scene of the emergency, and doctors and nurses who specialize in emergency care.

Prehospital emergency medical services are provided by emergency medical technicians (EMTs) trained to give care to accident victims and people with a sudden illness. The EMTs provide treatment until the person is transferred to the care of doctors and nurses in a hospital emergency department.

EMERGENCY MEDICAL TECHNICIANS

Certification skills and abilities for EMTs vary from state to state. In most states, there are three levels of training. The basic level is the EMT-A, which stands for emergency medical technician – ambulance. The next level is the EMT-I, for those medical technicians who undergo intermediate training. Finally, the EMT-P is the paramedic – the most highly skilled medical technician. Fewer than half the states designate two other categories called EMT-D (for ambulance personnel trained in defibrillation techniques – see page 130) and EMT-CC (for intermediate-level personnel trained in several critical care procedures).

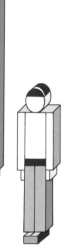
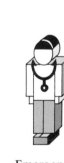
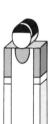

EMT-A	EMT-I	EMT-P	Emergency physicians	Emergency nurses
435,000	36,000	51,000	25,000	70,000

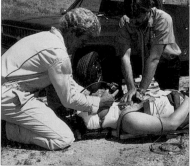
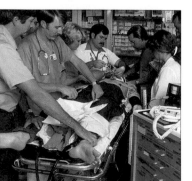

Responding to a medical emergency
EMTs begin evaluation and treatment at the scene of an emergency (far left). Once the ambulance arrives at the hospital, the staff of the emergency department take over the medical care of the patient (left).

Role of the EMTs

The EMT is responsible for the care of his or her ambulance and its equipment and must be certain that the medical supplies in the ambulance are fully stocked at all times. The EMT is trained to stabilize the patient's condition at the scene of the accident or medical emergency and to provide the necessary care until arrival at the hospital emergency department. The EMT gives the emergency department doctor or nurse a description of the accident or medical emergency, the patient's physical condition, and the treatment that has already been given.

AMBULANCES

The ambulance is designed to allow EMTs to provide medical care at the scene of an emergency and to transport an accident victim or person with a sudden illness to a hospital. Most counties or large cities have a system that determines the hospitals to which the patients are transported, based on the severity and type of injury or illness (see page 128).

A basic life-support ambulance carries the equipment necessary to give first-aid treatment, immobilize an injured arm, leg, or neck, and supply oxygen. In addition, an advanced life-support ambulance carries the equipment required for administering intravenous fluids and medication, heart monitoring, airway intubation, and defibrillation (see INSIDE AN AMBULANCE on page 126).

Since the early 1970s, two types of air ambulances – the helicopter and the airplane – have emerged as important components of emergency medical services. In some areas, helicopters are used to take accident victims to a hospital or to transfer patients from one hospital to another (see page 127). An airplane ambulance permits transport of patients over thousands of miles, but requires loading and unloading at an airport. This type of air ambulance is usually used to move patients whose conditions are stable.

WHAT HAPPENS WHEN YOU CALL AN EMERGENCY NUMBER?

In a medical emergency, call 911 (or the designated emergency number in your community) to contact the emergency medical services system. Tell the dispatcher the location of the emergency, how many people are injured, the types of injuries or illness, and the number of the telephone you are calling from. The dispatcher will send the appropriate emergency services to the scene.

1 You or another witness activates the emergency medical services system by calling 911.

2 The dispatcher calls for an ambulance, directs the EMTs to the scene, and tells them what type of injury or illness has occurred.

3 The dispatcher may also inform the police of the emergency.

4 In a major incident, the base communication hospital may contact nearby hospitals, warning them to expect injury victims.

5 The ambulance arrives at the scene. The EMTs communicate by radio with personnel in the designated emergency department and provide care to stabilize the patient's condition.

6 On the way to the nearest appropriate hospital (predetermined by the emergency medical services system), the EMTs monitor the patient's condition.

7 When the ambulance arrives at the hospital, the emergency department doctors and nurses take over care of the patient.

INSIDE AN AMBULANCE

An ambulance is designed to provide one of two levels of care – basic life support or advanced life support. The supplies and equipment an ambulance carries are determined by the level of care to be given. An advanced life-support ambulance is equipped to provide emergency medical care for victims of serious accidents and for critically ill people. This type of ambulance has all the first-aid supplies (such as splints, dressings, and painkillers) found on a basic life-support ambulance. In addition, it carries equipment – such as intravenous fluids, an electrocardiographic (ECG) monitor, a defibrillator, and a telemetry unit – needed to provide a more advanced level of care.

Stretcher
The stretcher (A) is one of the most basic components of any ambulance. It is adjustable and has wheels so that the patient can be easily moved in and out of the ambulance. During transportation to the hospital, the stretcher is secured into position within easy reach of equipment that the EMT may need to treat the patient.

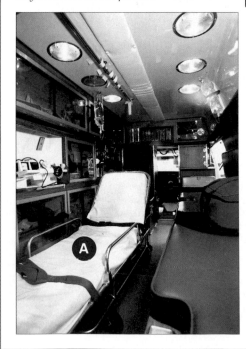

Defibrillator
The defibrillator (B) is used to reestablish a normal heart rhythm in a patient whose heart is beating irregularly or has stopped beating. A brief electric shock is administered to the heart with two paddles placed on the patient's chest.

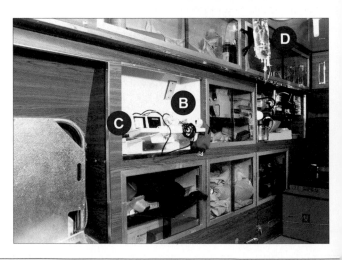

Telemetry unit
The telemetry unit (E) is a radio that allows voice communication and direct transmission of an ECG signal from the ambulance to the designated hospital. Doctors at the hospital give EMTs instructions for medical care. The EMTs are directed to the most appropriate hospital for treatment, and that hospital is informed of the patient's condition and estimated time of arrival.

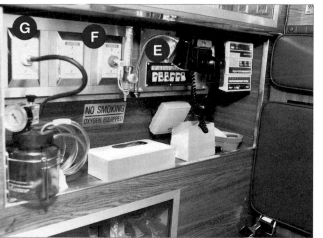

Oxygen equipment
Oxygen may be given to a patient who is having difficulty breathing. Oxygen is administered from an oxygen tank (F) into the patient's lungs through a face mask or tubing in the nose.

Suction equipment
The suction equipment (G) consists of a pump attached to a tube that can be inserted into the trachea (windpipe) or mouth to remove secretions (such as blood or vomit) that may interfere with breathing.

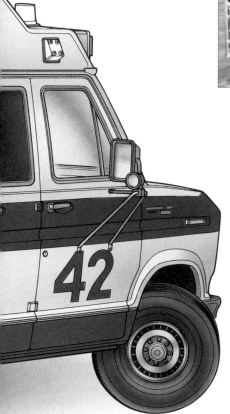

AIR AMBULANCES

Air ambulances can be particularly useful in rural areas, where advanced medical care is often not readily available. An air ambulance can transport a patient much more quickly than a ground ambulance – a helicopter air ambulance can travel at speeds of 120 to 180 miles per hour. It can also fly into otherwise inaccessible areas and land in confined spaces to reach accident victims.

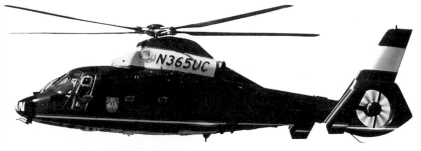

Intravenous drip
The intravenous drip (D) is used to infuse fluids and medications into the patient's bloodstream. The fluid flows from a plastic or glass container through tubing into a cannula (a small tube) that is inserted into a vein, often in the patient's forearm.

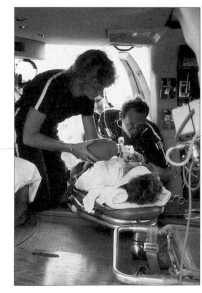

Inside the air ambulance
An air ambulance and its crew may be equipped to provide a higher level of medical care than an advanced life-support ground ambulance. Most commonly, the crew aboard a medical helicopter includes a nurse and a paramedic. Some aircraft are staffed by a nurse and a doctor. The crew ensures that the critically ill or injured person receives the most comprehensive medical care possible during the crucial period before and during transport to a hospital.

ECG monitor
The ECG equipment (C) can monitor the patient's heartbeat for any abnormal rhythms. The ECG signal can be transmitted via a telemetry unit (see above) to a hospital emergency department to produce a replica of the signals on the ECG monitor in the ambulance.

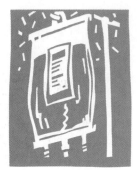

THE EMERGENCY DEPARTMENT

NEARLY 90 MILLION PEOPLE received medical care at hospital emergency departments in 1989. Only about 5 percent of the patients admitted to hospital emergency departments have a life-threatening injury or condition; 25 percent of patient visits are for noncritical emergencies and 70 percent are for nonemergencies.

There are currently more than 5,000 hospital emergency departments in the US. A state or local licensing agency categorizes hospitals according to their emergency and intensive care capabilities. Category 1 hospitals are able to offer the most comprehensive and advanced level of care. Hospitals in categories 2 and 3 can provide successively less advanced levels of care in their emergency departments and intensive care units. A category 4 hospital has a basic emergency department facility but does not have an intensive care unit. Many areas have designated specific hospital emergency departments as trauma centers, which are capable of providing advanced intensive trauma care 24 hours a day.

PATIENT CARE

The lives of thousands of people are saved every year by the treatment they receive in hospital emergency departments. The emergency department personnel assess the condition of each person and treat those with the greatest need first; this system is known as triage. Any illness or injury that interferes with breathing or circulation is treated immediately in the emergency department. Once any life-threatening conditions have been treated and stabilized, a severely injured or ill patient may have diagnostic tests and further treatment before being transferred to the intensive

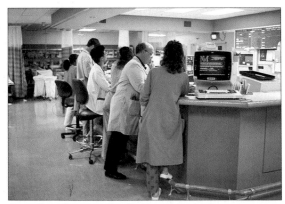

Coordinating care in the emergency department
Effective emergency care depends on good communications among all the personnel involved. In the emergency department shown above, the patient treatment areas are located around a central administration desk. Medications, computerized results from laboratory tests, patient records, posting of doctors' names who are on call, and other information essential to the care of the patients are kept in this area.

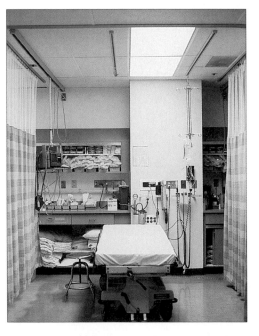

Patient treatment area
Most treatment areas in the emergency department are equipped for a wide range of emergencies. Equipment for suctioning fluids, measuring blood pressure, and supplying oxygen is mounted on the wall behind the bed. An electrocardiograph (ECG) monitor is on the left. The treatment area is stocked with basic supplies such as dressings and syringes. Other equipment, such as portable X-ray and ECG machines, are brought in as needed.

care unit or the operating room. Patients with less serious illnesses or injuries are treated and then may be sent home or admitted to the hospital for observation or further medical care.

TREATING BREATHING PROBLEMS

Patients with severe breathing difficulties are given immediate treatment in the emergency department. Lifesaving procedures to open the airway, such as a cricothyrotomy (see page 114), may be done after other methods of removing an airway obstruction have failed. Some people who are unable to breathe (for example, as a result of a drug overdose or a head injury) require intubation and mechanical ventilation (see below). Once the patient is breathing with assistance from the ventilator and all other conditions are stable, he or she may be taken to the intensive care unit for more treatment and monitoring or to the operating room if surgery is necessary.

MECHANICAL VENTILATION

Mechanical ventilation is required for patients who need assistance breathing as a result of illness or injury. The patient may be given a sedative or muscle relaxant; medical personnel then insert a laryngoscope into the patient's throat to allow examination of the vocal cords and upper part of the trachea (windpipe). A flexible tube, called an endotracheal tube, is then passed down the throat and between the vocal cords into the trachea – a procedure called airway intubation. The endotracheal tube is attached to the ventilator, which pumps air into the patient's lungs.

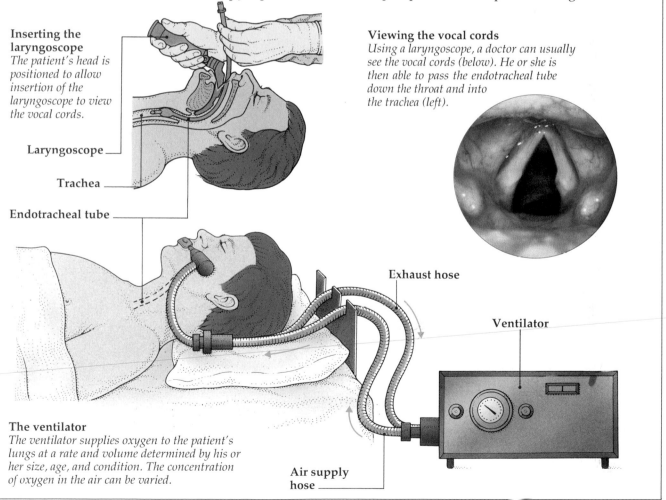

Inserting the laryngoscope
The patient's head is positioned to allow insertion of the laryngoscope to view the vocal cords.

Laryngoscope

Trachea

Endotracheal tube

Viewing the vocal cords
Using a laryngoscope, a doctor can usually see the vocal cords (below). He or she is then able to pass the endotracheal tube down the throat and into the trachea (left).

Exhaust hose

Ventilator

The ventilator
The ventilator supplies oxygen to the patient's lungs at a rate and volume determined by his or her size, age, and condition. The concentration of oxygen in the air can be varied.

Air supply hose

TREATING CARDIAC EMERGENCIES

A serious medical emergency such as cardiac arrest (cessation of the heart's pumping action) or major physical trauma requires intensive care. Most emergency departments have equipment to monitor and support vital body functions, such as the heartbeat and breathing.

After these vital functions are stabilized, the patient may be transferred to the cardiac or intensive care unit for further monitoring and treatment or to the operating room if surgery is necessary.

Monitoring the heartbeat

The electrodes of an electrocardiograph (ECG) are applied to a patient's skin to monitor the electrical activity of the heart. Abnormalities produce different patterns on the ECG, helping the doctor to diagnose a variety of heart rhythm disorders. If a patient's heart stops beating or beats very quickly or very slowly, an alarm on the ECG monitor rings to alert the staff.

Defibrillator
The paddles of the defibrillator are placed on the patient's chest. The buttons on both paddles are pressed simultaneously to deliver an electric shock to the heart. The resulting changes in heart rhythm are monitored on the ECG.

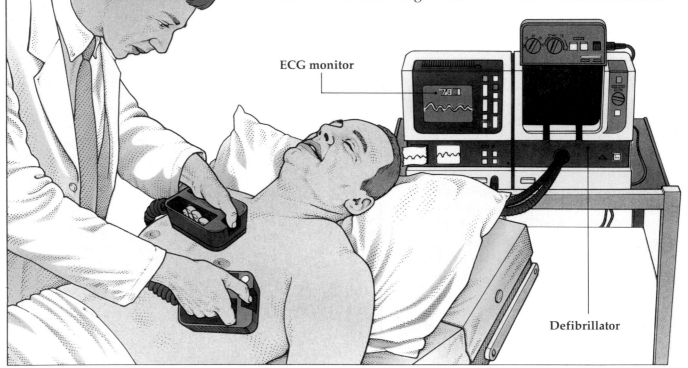

ECG monitor

Defibrillator

MONITORING THE HEART'S ELECTRICAL ACTIVITY

ECG monitoring
The ECG electrodes on the patient's chest sense the electrical activity of the heart. The pattern of the heart's electrical activity is shown on a screen and recorded on a moving strip of paper.

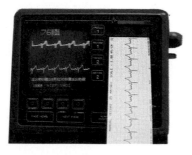

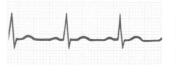

Normal ECG recording
The normal electrical activity of a heart is indicated by the regularly repeated and distinctive pattern shown on this ECG recording.

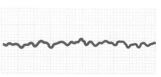

Ventricular fibrillation
In this type of abnormal heart rhythm, the ventricles quiver without pumping blood. The ECG shows no distinct shape – only irregular, rapid waves.

Abnormal heartbeat

Ventricular fibrillation is a condition in which the ventricles of the heart beat in a rapid, irregular pattern. This type of abnormal heartbeat can be fatal because blood is not effectively pumped around the body. The defibrillator (see page 130), a machine that delivers an electric shock to the heart, can be used to convert an abnormal heart rhythm to a normal one. If the normal rhythm is not restored after defibrillation, the procedure may be repeated using a more powerful shock.

The heartbeat is controlled by tissues in the heart that distribute impulses to the muscles of the heart, causing them to contract. Failure of this natural pacemaking mechanism leads to arrhythmias (irregular heartbeat). Artificial pacemakers are used to supply electrical impulses to the heart muscle to maintain the heartbeat at an efficient rate. In the emergency department, one of three types of temporary pacemakers (see right) may be used – transvenous (inserted through a vein into the heart), transthoracic (inserted through the chest wall into the heart), or transcutaneous (applied to the chest). A temporary pacemaker can be removed when the heart no longer needs artificial pacing or may be replaced by a permanent pacemaker.

Cardiac arrest

After evaluating the airway and breathing pattern of a patient with possible cardiac arrest (cessation of the heart's pumping action), the doctor or nurse checks for a pulse. If there is no pulse, the medical team begins cardiopulmonary resuscitation immediately to help restore breathing and circulation. A defibrillator may be used to deliver a brief electric shock to the heart. The procedure may be repeated several times in conjunction with giving drugs that stimulate or stabilize the activity of the heart. Once the heartbeat is reestablished, the patient is transferred to the intensive care unit for monitoring and further treatment.

TEMPORARY PACEMAKERS

Artificial pacemakers are devices used to reestablish and maintain the heart's normal rate and rhythm. In the emergency department, a temporary pacemaker may be used if a patient's heart begins to beat too slowly or irregularly.

Inserting a transvenous pacemaker
A hollow needle (called a catheter) is inserted into a vein in the patient's neck. The pacemaker wire is guided into the hollow needle and moved through the vein until the electrode at the end of the wire is inside the heart. The free end of the wire is connected to the pacemaker, which discharges impulses as needed to stimulate the heart to beat.

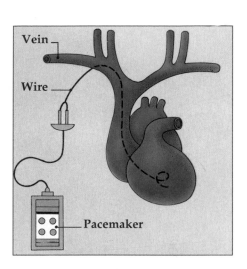

Inserting a transthoracic pacemaker
A transthoracic pacemaker is inserted directly through the chest wall into the heart. A hollow needle is inserted into one of the chambers of the heart, and the pacemaker wire is guided through the needle into the heart. The needle is then removed, and the wire is attached to the pacemaker, which sends impulses as needed to stimulate the heart to beat.

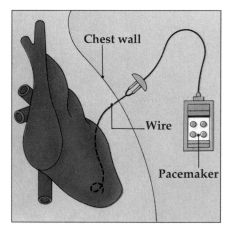

Applying a transcutaneous pacemaker
External pacemaker pads are placed on the patient's chest, over the heart (as shown on the mannequin at right), and on the patient's back, between the shoulder blades. The pads are connected to a monitor that senses the patient's heart rate. When the heart rate slows, the pacemaker pads emit an impulse that stimulates the heart to beat.

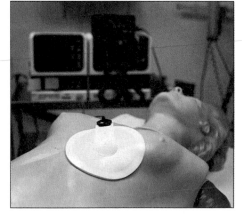

TREATING POISONING

Victims of poisoning or drug overdose receive immediate medical attention in the emergency department. If the person is conscious, the doctor asks him or her what substance was taken and how long ago. A poison may remain in the stomach for 4 hours or more.

Treatment is given to prevent absorption of the poison into the bloodstream. Two methods may be used to remove substances from the stomach – pumping the stomach (see right) and giving an emetic. An emetic is a substance that induces vomiting, either by stimulating the part of the brain that controls vomiting or by irritating the lining of the stomach. The most commonly used emetic is syrup of ipecac. Emetics are not used when the person is unconscious or nearly unconscious because the person may inhale vomit into the lungs. Activated charcoal is often given after the stomach has been emptied to soak up any remaining poisons before they can be absorbed by the gastrointestinal tract.

Corrosive poisons

If a person has swallowed corrosive poison, neither a stomach pumping procedure nor an emetic is appropriate. The tube used to pump the stomach can perforate the stomach if its wall has been weakened by the poison. If the person vomits, the esophagus may be damaged more as the corrosive substance moves back up to the mouth. Instead, the doctor may administer a substance that dilutes the poison in the person's stomach. Corrosive acids or alkalis may be diluted with large amounts of water or milk.

Follow-up treatment

Follow-up treatment for poisoning depends on the type of poison and the circumstances of the poisoning. Some poisons have an antidote that is given to counter the effects of any of the poison that has been absorbed.

PUMPING THE STOMACH

Gastric lavage, or pumping the stomach, is used to remove a poison from the stomach before the body can absorb it. The doctor or nurse inserts a tube (called an orogastric tube) down the esophagus into the stomach. Water or sterile fluids flow into the stomach through this tube. After 2 to 3 minutes the diluted contents of the stomach are suctioned out.

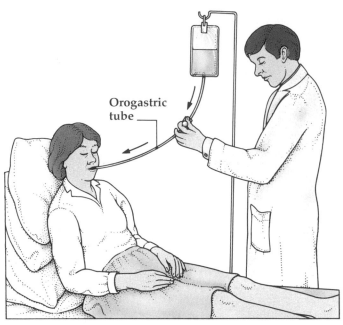

Conscious patient
A conscious patient having gastric lavage may be lying on his or her side with feet elevated 6 to 12 inches or may be seated at a 45- to 90-degree angle. The semireclining position helps prevent inhalation of the fluid into the lungs.

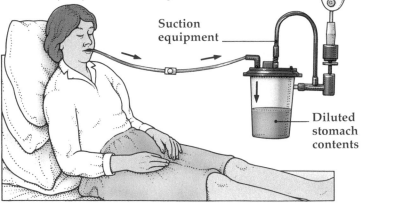

Suction equipment

Diluted stomach contents

Stomach contents
The wash-out procedure is repeated until the stomach contents appear clear. If the type of poison is not known, a sample from the first wash-out procedure may be analyzed.

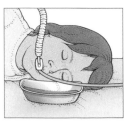

Unconscious patient
An unconscious patient undergoing gastric lavage has an endotracheal tube inserted into the windpipe to prevent fluid from the stomach from entering the lungs.

CLEANING AND SUTURING WOUNDS

Wounds are the most common type of injury treated in hospital emergency departments. If a wound is still bleeding, direct pressure is applied to the wound to stop the flow of blood. The wound is examined, cleaned with antiseptic, and rinsed with sterile fluids. If necessary, the edges of the wound are then sutured (stitched) together.

Removing objects from a wound
When a wound contains foreign objects, such as gravel embedded over a large area, it may require cleaning while the patient is sedated in the emergency department or under general anesthesia in the operating room.

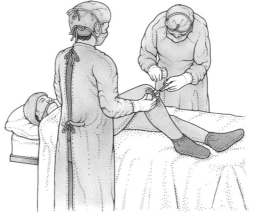

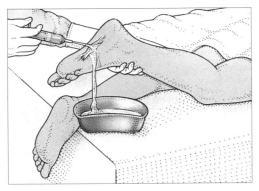

Cleaning a wound
After foreign objects or dead tissue is removed from a wound, it must be thoroughly cleaned to minimize the possibility of infection. The wound may be cleaned by washing it repeatedly with a medicated or sterile solution.

Closing wounds
If a wound is shallow and not gaping, adhesive strips or butterfly bandages can be used to hold the edges together. If a wound is deep, severed nerves and tendons may have to be sewn together before the wound is closed with sutures. Sometimes, the wound is stitched temporarily until surgery can be performed to repair the tendons and nerves.

Adhesive tapes
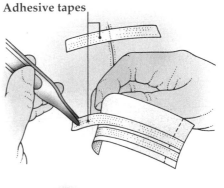

SUTURES

In the emergency department, the doctor chooses a suture (stitch) material and technique according to the size and depth of the wound. Types of suture materials include catgut (which is made from sheep's intestines), linen, silk, or synthetic thread (such as nylon). An anesthetic is usually injected into and around the wound before it is stitched. In some emergency departments, staples are used to close certain types of wounds.

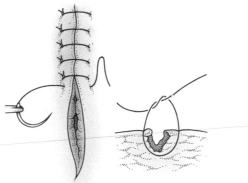

Interrupted sutures
The interrupted suture is the type of stitch most commonly used for closing wounds. The doctor passes the needle into the skin, through the full depth of the wound, and out the other side. Each stitch is then knotted on one side of the wound.

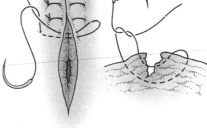

Mattress sutures
Mattress sutures are used for deep wounds. Each stitch passes through the wound twice, first near the surface of the wound and then deeper into the wound. Each stitch is knotted on one side of the wound.

DISSOLVABLE SUTURES
The dissolvable suture (stitch), usually made of catgut, may be used to sew up a cut. These sutures are not removed, but rather are dissolved by enzymes in the body over a period of time. Dissolvable sutures are often used in the mouth or deep inside a wound if muscles or other tissues must be held together beneath the skin. These types of sutures are not usually used to sew the outer skin layer together.

EMERGENCY SYMPTOMS

Some symptoms, such as fever, headache, and nausea, are very common and may or may not indicate a serious medical condition. Other symptoms, such as sudden chest pain or vomiting blood, are usually signals of a serious medical condition. Being able to recognize symptoms and relate the symptoms to specific injuries and conditions is a very important part of providing the appropriate first-aid treatment. Whatever the symptom, if it is severe or prolonged get medical help immediately.

Your body has a number of systems that work together to keep it functioning efficiently. This section describes symptoms produced by the various body systems that require prompt medical attention.

CARDIOVASCULAR SYMPTOMS

The cardiovascular system consists of the heart and blood vessels. Blood is pumped by the heart and circulated through the blood vessels to deliver oxygen to, and remove carbon dioxide from, the cells of your body. Medical emergencies can occur when an injury or illness interferes with the normal function of this system.

Chest pain

Chest pain can signal a life-threatening condition, such as a heart attack (see page 49) or pulmonary embolism (see below). If a person has sudden, severe chest pain, call for emergency medical help. Make the person comfortable in a sitting or semireclining position – the person should not lie down flat if it makes breathing more difficult. Loosen tight clothing. Restore breathing and circulation if necessary (see page 45).

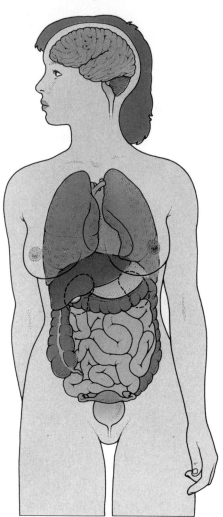

Your body systems
Good health demands efficient interaction of your body systems. A disorder of or injury to one or more of these systems disrupts this critical interaction, causing a variety of emergency symptoms.

Pulmonary embolism
A sharp, stabbing chest pain accompanied by breathlessness, fainting, or blood in the sputum may indicate a pulmonary embolism – the blockage of a blood vessel in the lungs by a blood clot.

Clot

Area lacking
blood supply

Palpitations

Palpitations (awareness of your heartbeat) are usually not serious; they may be felt after strenuous exercise or a severe scare, when the heart is beating harder and faster than normal. Palpitations felt at rest may indicate anxiety or a disorder that is causing the heart to beat irregularly, very fast, or very slowly. If palpitations result in breathlessness, chest pain, or fainting, call for medical help immediately. Keep the person comfortable and loosen tight clothing. Restore breathing and circulation if necessary (see page 45).

Leg pain

In some cases, leg pain that has no obvious external cause can indicate a condition that requires immediate treatment by a doctor. Such conditions include an insufficient supply of blood to the leg or a blood clot in one of the deep veins in the leg (see right). If a person experiences a sudden pain in his or her leg, have the person lie down and rest the leg. Call a doctor as soon as possible.

RESPIRATORY SYMPTOMS

The respiratory system consists of the lungs and the passages through which air enters the lungs. Oxygen is inhaled into the lungs and absorbed into the blood; the waste product carbon dioxide is transferred from the blood to the lungs and exhaled. It is vital to recognize and treat respiratory emergencies immediately because, if breathing stops, brain damage and death may occur as a result of the lack of oxygen.

Breathing problems

Breathing problems can be caused by a wide variety of medical conditions. Possible causes of breathing difficulty include a pneumothorax (see page 80), an asthma attack (see page 112), pulmonary edema (see page 113), choking (see page 114), anaphylactic shock (see page 117), pneumonia (inflammation of the lungs caused by an infection), or respiratory failure (in which carbon dioxide levels build up in the blood and oxygen levels fall). A prolonged interruption of breathing can lead to cyanosis, a condition in which the lips and skin under the nails become blue as a result of a lack of oxygen. If cyanosis develops, immediate medical treatment is critical.

A person who is having difficulty breathing needs to see a doctor immediately; take the person to the nearest hospital emergency department or call an ambulance. If an object is obstructing the airway, at-

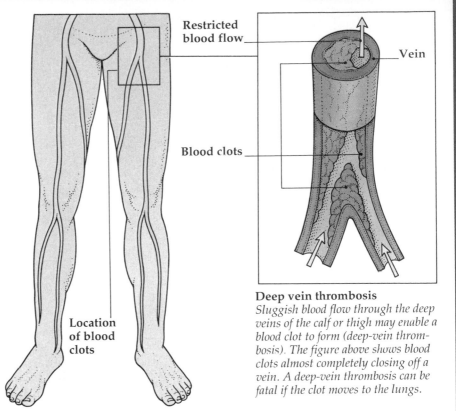

Location of blood clots

Restricted blood flow

Vein

Blood clots

Deep vein thrombosis
Sluggish blood flow through the deep veins of the calf or thigh may enable a blood clot to form (deep-vein thrombosis). The figure above shows blood clots almost completely closing off a vein. A deep-vein thrombosis can be fatal if the clot moves to the lungs.

tempt to clear the airway immediately (see page 52). Keep the person comfortable and sitting up to help make his or her breathing easier. If the person stops breathing, perform artificial ventilation immediately (see page 47). If the person's heart stops beating, start cardiopulmonary resuscitation (see page 50).

Blood in the sputum

Coughing up blood is an extremely alarming experience; tell your doctor as soon as you can. Although blood in the sputum may be a sign of bronchitis, it may also be a sign of a more serious condition such as pulmonary embolism (see page 134), pneumonia (inflammation of the lungs caused by an infection), or pulmonary edema (see page 113).

Asthma attacks
If difficulty breathing occurs when a person exhales, and is accompanied by a wheezing or whistling sound, the cause of the breathing difficulty may be an asthma attack. In most cases an asthma attack can be effectively treated by inhaling a bronchodilator drug, which widens the airways in the lungs. A severe asthma attack may require hospitalization.

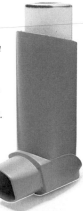

First aid for vomiting blood
Vomiting large quantities of blood may cause physical collapse. Call for medical help immediately. If a person is dizzy or faints, lay the person on his or her side to prevent choking on the vomit.

DIGESTIVE SYMPTOMS

The digestive system consists of the digestive tract (the mouth, esophagus, stomach, small intestine, large intestine, and anus) and the liver, gallbladder, and pancreas. Symptoms of digestive problems are often general, making it difficult to determine the specific type of disorder on the basis of symptoms alone.

Vomiting blood
Vomiting blood requires emergency treatment. Possible causes of vomiting blood include a bleeding peptic ulcer (see below), erosion of the stomach lining, esophagitis (inflammation of the esophagus), ruptured veins in the esophagus, or a tear at the lower end of the esophagus caused by very strenuous vomiting.

If a person is vomiting blood, call for medical help immediately. Do not allow the person to eat or drink or take any medication. Make the person as comfortable as possible in a sitting position. If the person feels dizzy or faint, have the person lie on his or her side (see above).

Blood in stools
Blood in stools indicates bleeding in the gastrointestinal tract. If you see blood in your stools, call your doctor as soon as possible. Passing large quantities of red blood or dark blood in the stools is an emergency; go to the nearest hospital. Blood in the stools may be caused by dilated veins in the walls of the esophagus that have ruptured, peptic ulcers (see left), erosion of the stomach lining, and Crohn's disease and ulcerative colitis (the two most common inflammatory bowel diseases).

Diarrhea and vomiting
Diarrhea or vomiting that lasts for more than 24 hours can lead to dehydration, a condition caused by the loss of an excessive amount of fluid from the body (see right); call your doctor. Vomiting that occurs after an accident may be caused by a head or abdominal injury. Call an ambulance. Keep the person lying down until medical help arrives.

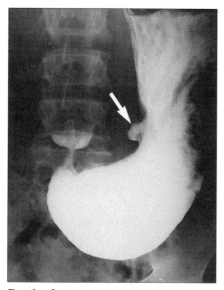

Peptic ulcer
A bleeding peptic ulcer is a common cause of blood in vomit or stools. The X-ray above shows a large ulcer in the stomach. Symptoms of a bleeding peptic ulcer may include sudden weakness, fainting, and, in severe cases, collapse.

Self-help for diarrhea and vomiting
To help prevent dehydration, take sips of water, diluted fruit juice, or tea. If you are vomiting, do not drink more than 2 ounces of fluid every 30 minutes until your nausea goes away. Packets of premixed ingredients (available from your pharmacist) can be added to water to promote rehydration.

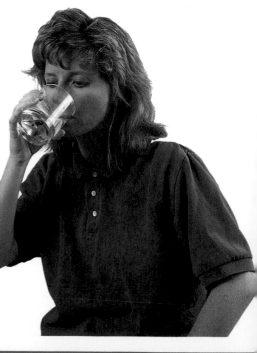

CAUSES OF ABDOMINAL PAIN

There are hundreds of causes of abdominal pain. In some cases, abdominal pain indicates a serious condition that requires medical attention. If you have persistent abdominal pain, call your doctor immediately. Never give laxatives, enemas, medications, food, or liquids to a person with abdominal pain without a doctor's advice.

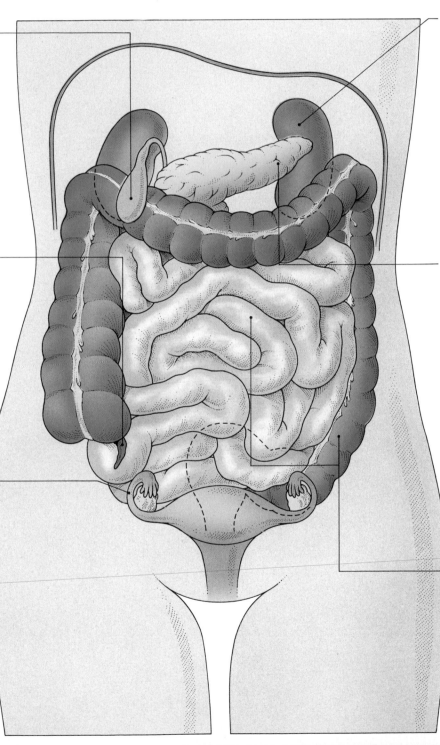

Inflammation of the gallbladder
Inflammation of the gallbladder usually causes pain in the upper right part of the abdomen. The pain often radiates around or into the back, just below the right shoulder blade. Fever, nausea, and vomiting may also occur.

Appendicitis
Appendicitis (inflammation of the appendix) usually causes pain and tenderness in the lower right side of the abdomen. Other symptoms and signs may include constipation, fever, nausea, and vomiting.

Ectopic (tubal) pregnancy
A ruptured ectopic pregnancy is an emergency that requires immediate medical attention. Symptoms may include moderate or severe pain on one side of the lower part of the abdomen, vaginal bleeding (see VAGINAL BLEEDING on page 141), dizziness, abnormal paleness, sweating, and rapid pulse.

Kidney stone
A kidney stone forms when substances in the urine crystallize and form a hard deposit. Symptoms are severe pain in the side or back that radiates to the groin, usually accompanied by sweating, abnormal paleness, nausea, and vomiting.

Pancreatitis
Pancreatitis (inflammation of the pancreas) can cause a sudden pain in the upper part of the abdomen. The pain may be aggravated by any movement. Other symptoms and signs may include sweating, back pain, nausea, vomiting, a rapid pulse, and collapse.

Bowel obstruction
An obstruction of the bowel causes pain that may become increasingly severe and is accompanied by distention of the abdomen, nausea, vomiting, and inability to pass gas.

NERVOUS SYSTEM SYMPTOMS

The nervous system functions as the body's control, communications, and information processing system. Nerve pathways throughout the body send information to the brain and carry back signals that control voluntary and involuntary responses. Disorders of the nervous system may be caused by damage or dysfunction of a component of the system or by impairment of the system's sensory, analytical, memory, or motor functions.

Severe headache and stiff neck

A severe headache on one side of your head accompanied by disturbances of vision, nausea, and vomiting may be a migraine (see below). If you have not previously had migraine headaches, you should call your doctor as soon as possible. If a person with a headache shows any change in his or her level of consciousness, call for medical help immediately. A headache may also be caused by a subdural hemorrhage (see page 70) or glaucoma. A severe headache accompanied by a stiff neck may be caused by meningitis, subarachnoid hemorrhage (see page 70), or a head or neck injury (see page 72). If a head or neck injury has

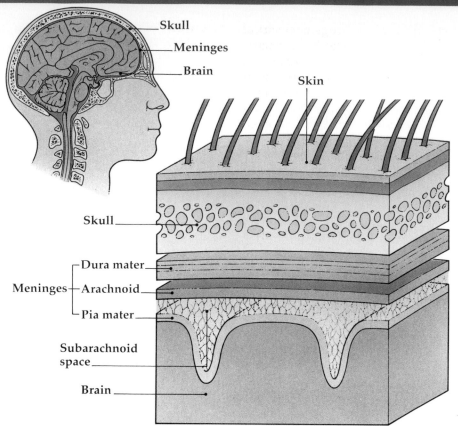

Meningitis
Meningitis is inflammation of the membranes (called the meninges) that cover the brain and spinal cord – usually as the result of an infection. The meninges may become infected by organisms carried in the bloodstream or that have penetrated the skull through a fracture or spread from an infected ear or sinus. Symptoms may include severe headache, fever, nausea and vomiting, and a stiff neck. In most cases, meningitis is life-threatening. See your doctor immediately.

occurred, immobilize the person's head and neck (see page 73) and call for emergency medical help.

A severe headache in a pregnant woman may be a symptom of preeclampsia, a serious condition in which high blood pressure, fluid retention, and proteinuria (protein in the urine) develop in the second half of pregnancy. Preeclampsia requires emergency treatment by a doctor.

Seizures
Although seizures appear alarming, most people recover from them within a few minutes. Seizures may occur with epilepsy, a head injury, poisoning, heat stroke, high fever,

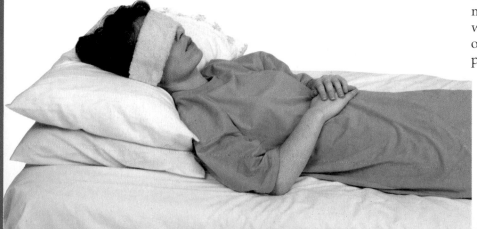

Self-help for severe headache
If you have a severe headache and do not have a history of migraines, call your doctor as soon as possible. Most headaches are caused by tension and can usually be relieved by aspirin and rest. Turn off the lights if they hurt your eyes, place a damp cloth over your forehead, and sit or lie in a comfortable position.

withdrawal from drugs, or electrical shock. A person who has a seizure needs prompt medical attention. A person with a known seizure disorder needs emergency treatment if the seizure lasts longer than 2 minutes, if one seizure follows another, or if the person's confusion or disorientation persists.

Fainting

Fainting that follows anxiety or stress is usually not a life-threatening emergency (see page 57). Fainting that requires immediate medical attention may be caused by the sudden onset of irregular heartbeats (see PALPITATIONS on page 134), dehydration, severe bleeding, or shock.

If a person feels faint, have the person lie down and elevate his or her feet. If a person faints, maintain an open airway (see page 45) and loosen tight clothing, especially around the neck. If the person who has fainted vomits, place the person on his or her side or turn the head to one side. Bathe the person's face with cool water and check for injuries

caused by falling. Do not give the person anything to drink unless he or she seems fully recovered. Seek prompt medical attention.

Confusion

The sudden onset of confusion and drowsiness requires immediate medical help. If these symptoms occur with paralysis, they may indicate a stroke. A head injury (see page 70), severe infection, diabetic ketoacidosis (very high levels of sugar and acid in the blood) or insulin shock (a very low level of sugar in the

blood), some medications, or abuse of alcohol or other drugs may also cause confusion and drowsiness (see LOSS OF CONSCIOUSNESS on page 140).

If a person seems confused and may have had a stroke or head injury, get medical help immediately. If the person has a possible head injury, do not move his or her neck. Keep the person comfortable and apply cold cloths to the head. Do not

First aid for faintness
A person who feels faint should lie down with his or her legs elevated 8 to 12 inches (below). The person may also sit down and slowly bend forward so that his or her head is between the knees (right); move any objects out of the person's way to prevent injury if the person falls.

RECOGNIZING A SEIZURE

A person having a seizure often utters a short cry or scream and his or her muscles become rigid. This is followed by jerking, twisting movements. Breathing may temporarily stop, the lips may become blue, and the eyes may roll upward. The person may drool or lose bowel or bladder control. After the seizure has stopped, the person is often unresponsive, drowsy, and confused.

First aid for seizures
If a person has a seizure, gently lay him or her down. Loosen tight clothing around the neck. Move any objects that the person may strike. If the person stops breathing, start artificial ventilation (see page 47) after the seizure has stopped. Do not interfere with the person's movements or place anything in his or her mouth. After the seizure has stopped, keep the person lying on his or her side to prevent choking. Call for medical help. Check for injuries, such as bleeding, and stay with the person until medical help arrives.

give the person anything to eat or drink (to prevent choking). Restore breathing and circulation if necessary (see page 45).

Psychotic or aggressive behavior

Psychotic or aggressive behavior may result from schizophrenia or other types of mental illness, a head injury (see CONFUSION on page 139), diabetic ketoacidosis (very high levels of sugar and acid in the blood), or abuse of alcohol or other drugs. Call your local emergency services number immediately. If necessary, and only if approaching the person will not endanger your safety, try to prevent the person from harming himself or herself.

Loss of consciousness

A person who loses consciousness needs medical attention immediately. A severe heart attack (see CHEST PAIN on page 134), a stroke or head injury (see CONFUSION on page 139), severe alcohol or other drug abuse, choking or anaphylactic shock (see BREATHING PROBLEMS on page 135), or diabetic insulin shock (a very low level of sugar in the blood) may cause unconsciousness.

A person who is unconscious and breathing should be kept lying down; maintain an open airway and loosen any tight clothing. Check for possible causes of unconsciousness, such as bleeding or a head injury. If the cause of the unconsciousness is unknown, always suspect a head, neck, or back injury and do not move the person except to maintain an open airway. If the person is not breathing, restore breathing and circulation if necessary (see page 45).

Place a person who is unconscious and begins vomiting on his or her side, with the head slightly lower than the rest of the body, to prevent choking. Never leave the person alone, do not give food or liquids, and keep the person comfortable until medical help arrives.

GENITOURINARY SYMPTOMS

The term "genitourinary" includes the urinary system (consisting of the kidneys, ureters, bladder, and urethra) and the reproductive system.

Inability to pass urine

Inability to urinate is a painful and distressing condition and requires prompt medical help. The condition may be caused by an infection of the urinary tract or by an enlarged prostate gland (see below).

If a person is unable to urinate, call his or her doctor or take the person to the nearest hospital. Do not give the person any liquids; this will increase the urge to urinate. Reassurance is important because anxiety or panic often makes the painful symptoms worse.

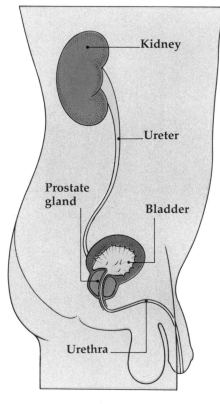

Enlarged prostate gland
An enlarged prostate gland is a common occurrence in older men. Enlargement of the prostate gland may lead to an inability to urinate. Surgery may be required.

Blood in the urine

Blood in the urine may be caused by an infection in the kidneys or throughout the urinary tract, stones in the kidneys or the bladder, injury, tumors in the urinary or reproductive system, or a variety of inflammatory conditions. Call your doctor immediately. Red blood cells may be present in the urine even though the urine does not appear red.

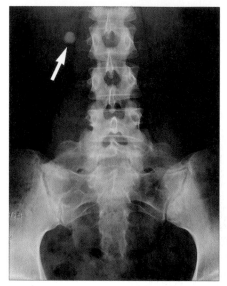

Blood in the urine
Blood in the urine may be caused by a kidney stone. In the X-ray above, a stone has moved from the kidney and is blocking the ureter, causing bleeding from the blood vessels in the ureter. The X-ray below shows a bladder with two tumors (arrows). Such cancers cause bleeding into the urine by damaging the walls of the blood vessels in the bladder.

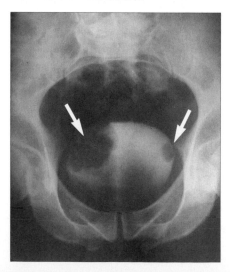

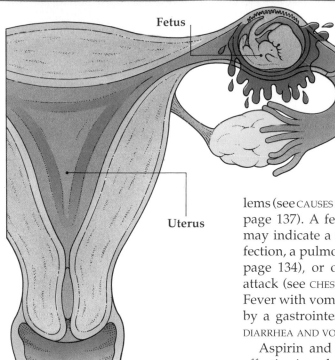

Fetus

Fallopian tube

Uterus

Ruptured ectopic (tubal) pregnancy

An ectopic pregnancy develops outside the uterus, usually in a fallopian tube. As the embryo grows, it becomes too large for the fallopian tube and causes the tube to rupture. A ruptured fallopian tube requires immediate surgery because excessive bleeding into the abdomen can occur, leading to shock and death.

Vaginal bleeding

Heavy vaginal bleeding is a medical emergency in a pregnant woman. Vaginal bleeding may be caused by a ruptured ectopic pregnancy (see above) or by a possible or actual miscarriage. Heavy vaginal bleeding in the middle to late stages of pregnancy often reflects serious complications and can be life-threatening for both the woman and fetus.

If you are pregnant and have any vaginal bleeding, call your doctor or go to the nearest hospital emergency department immediately. Save any tissue or blood clots that you pass so that they can be examined.

FEVER

While a fever is usually associated with viral infections, fever may also indicate a medical emergency. Heat stroke (with body temperatures above 104°F) can be fatal and requires immediate medical attention. Fever and severe head and neck ache may be caused by meningitis (see MENINGITIS on page 138). Fever accompanied by abdominal pain can indicate appendicitis or other prob-

lems (see CAUSES OF ABDOMINAL PAIN on page 137). A fever with chest pain may indicate a respiratory tract infection, a pulmonary embolism (see page 134), or occasionally a heart attack (see CHEST PAIN on page 134). Fever with vomiting may be caused by a gastrointestinal infection (see DIARRHEA AND VOMITING on page 136).

Aspirin and acetaminophen are effective in reducing a fever (do not give aspirin to children or teenagers). Call your doctor if a fever persists or is accompanied by other symptoms.

Acute glaucoma
Acute glaucoma is a condition in which the pressure of fluid in the eye increases. Symptoms are severe pain in and above the eye, a dilated pupil, a hazy cornea, and nausea and vomiting. Increased pressure may be caused by a blocked drainage channel between the iris and the back of the cornea (right), which may compress and damage the blood vessels and nerve fibers of the eye, leading to loss of vision.

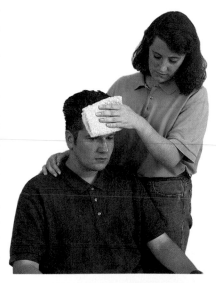

LOSS OF VISION

Loss of sight may be caused by several medical conditions, including a detached retina, acute glaucoma, injury to the eye, a sharp object that penetrates the eye, severe bacterial or viral infection, or closure of an artery or vein in the retina. If you have any loss of vision or blurring of vision in one or both eyes, talk to your doctor immediately. Sudden, unexpected loss of vision in one eye may indicate the beginning of a stroke.

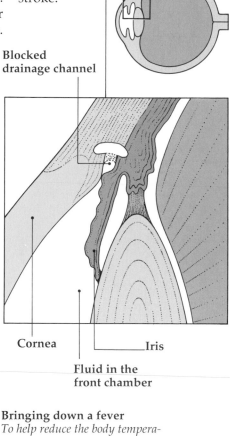

Blocked drainage channel

Cornea

Iris

Fluid in the front chamber

Bringing down a fever
To help reduce the body temperature of a person with a fever, move the person into a cool environment, remove heavy clothing, and sponge his or her forehead with lukewarm water.

Photograph sources:
Ardea London Ltd 96 (bottom left); 96
    (center); 117 (top right)
Audio-Visual Services 29
St. Bartholomew's Medical Picture Library
    103 (bottom left); 140
Bubbles Photo Library 24
Bruce Coleman Ltd 95; 96 (center left)
Dr S. Gwyther 136 (bottom left)
The Image Bank 9; 19; 30; 32 (bottom left);
    33 (top right); 33 (center right); 101
    (bottom right); 105 (center); 124
Institute of Orthopaedics 74
National Medical Slide Bank, UK 77
NHPA 118 (center right)
Oxford Scientific Films, Kathie Atkinson
    2 (top left) and 117 (top center); John
    Cooke 116 (center); James H.
    Robinson 116 (center right); Michael
    Sogden 118 (bottom left)

Pictures Colour Library 32 (top left); 33
    (bottom left)
Science Photo Library 55; 129
A.C. Scott, Central Veterinary Laboratory
    94 (bottom left)
Tony Stone Worldwide 31; 32/33 (center);
    64; 93 (top right); 105 (bottom)
Sygma Ltd 114 (bottom)
Zefa Picture Library 7; 20 (center); 33 (bot-
    tom right); 35; 61; 123
Front cover photograph:
© Duncan/Medical Images Inc.

Commissioned photography:
Susannah Price
Clive Streeter   Jim Ziv

The safety poster on page 28 was
reproduced with permission from
the National Safety Council.

Illustrators:
Russell Barnet   John Woodcock
Andrew Bezear
Joanna Cameron   **Airbrushing:**
Karen Cochrane   Paul Desmond
David Fathers   Roy Flooks
Tony Graham   Janos Marffy
Andrew Green
Kevin Marks   **Index:**
Philip Wilson   Sue Bosanko

Reader's Digest Fund for the Blind is
publisher of the Large-Type Edition of
Reader's Digest. For subscription information about this magazine, please
contact Reader's Digest Fund for the
Blind, Inc., Dept. 250, Pleasantville, N.Y.
10570.